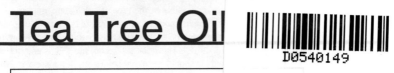

Tea Tree Oil

NATURE'S MIRACLE HEALER

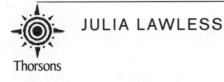

JULIA LAWLESS

Thorsons

While the authors of this work have made every effort to ensure that the information contained in this book is as accurate and up to date as possible at the time of publication, medical and pharmaceutical knowledge is constantly changing and the application of it to particular circumstances depends on many factors. Therefore it is recommended that readers always consult a qualified medical specialist for individual advice. This book should not be used as an alternative to seeking specialist medical advice, which should be sought before any action is taken. The author and publishers cannot be held responsible for any errors and omissions that may be found in the text, or any actions that may be taken by a reader as a result of any reliance on the information contained in the text, which is taken entirely at the reader's own risk.

Thorsons
An Imprint of HarperCollins*Publishers*
77–85 Fulham Palace Road,
Hammersmith, London W6 8JB

The Thorsons website address is: www.thorsons.com

Published by Thorsons 1994
This edition published by Thorsons 2001

10 9 8 7 6 5 4 3 2 1

© Julia Lawless 1994 and 2001

Julia Lawless asserts the moral right
to be identified as the author of this work

A catalogue record for this book
is available from the British Library

ISBN 0 00 711070 7

Printed in Great Britain by
Martins the Printers Limited, Berwick Upon Tweed

Thorsons
Directions for life

Dedicated to
ALEX AND CHIARA

OTHER BOOKS BY JULIA LAWLESS:

Aromatherapy and the Mind
The Complete Illustrated Guide to Aromatherapy
Home Aromatherapy
The Illustrated Encyclopedia of Essential Oils
Aloe Vera
Lavender Oil

About the Author

Having been brought up in a family with a strong herbal tradition, Julia Lawless has had an interest in aromatic plants ever since she was a child. Her Finnish mother, a biochemist, was involved in the research of aromatic oils and subsequently established her own essential oil company, Aqua Oleum. In 1983 Julia took over responsibility for the formulation of natural aromatic products for the family business. Julia has also studied Western and Tibetan herbal medicine and is a qualified aromatherapist, as well as being a passionate gardener.

Highly respected in her field, Julia has lectured internationally on aromatic plants and oils, appearing both on radio and television. She is the author of several books on aromatic plants and their uses, including the best-selling manuals *The Illustrated Encyclopedia of Essential Oils* and *The Complete Illustrated Guide to Aromatherapy*. She currently divides her time between London and Gloucestershire, where she has designed her own aromatherapy garden.

Contents

TEA TREE OIL

Acknowledgements	ix
Tea Tree Oil – An Introduction	xi

Part One: Tea Tree's Medical and Historical Background   1

Native Folk Remedy of the Australian Aborigines	3
Early Medical Research Reports	8
Evidence Obtained from Later Clinical Studies	12
Production, Chemical Composition and Quality Control	17
A Summary of the Properties and Applications of Tea Tree Oil	23
Methods of Use, Safety Data and Storage Precautions	27

Part Two: A–Z of Health Care Applications   33

Acne & spots; arthritis & gout; athlete's foot; balanitis; barber's rash; boils and abscesses; bronchitis; bumps & bruises; burns; candida; carbuncles; chickenpox; chilblains; colds; cold sores; corns; coughs; cracked skin; cradle cap; cuts & wounds; cystitis & urethritis;

dandruff; dermatitis & eczema; dhobi itch; disinfectant uses; fever; flu; genital herpes; hair care; hives (nettle rash); immune system, to strengthen; impetigo; insect bites & stings; leucorrhoea & pruritis; lice (pediculosis); measles; mouth & gum infections; muscular aches & pains; nappy rash; paronychia; pets & animal care; psoriasis; rheumatism; ringworm; scabies; sinusitis; skin care; sore throat; splinters, infected; sunburn; sweaty feet; thrush; ticks & leeches; ulcers, varicose & tropical; warts & veruccae; zona (shingles).

Part Three: Further Information   97

    Other Essential Oils from the Tea Tree Group   99

    The Constituents of Tea Tree Oil   101

    References   103

    Bibliography   108

    Useful Addresses   113

    Index   117

Acknowledgements

TEA TREE OIL

I would especially like to thank the following people who have helped to bring this book to fruition in a variety of ways: John Black, for his valuable expertise and for providing technical information; Cara Denman for her guidance; Jane Graham-Maw and those at Thorsons for their sympathetic approach to the project; Len Smith for his editorial notes and suggestions; and last but not least, my husband Alec and daughter Natasha for their constant support.

I would also like to thank the *Jour. Agric. Food Chem.* for their kind permission to reprint the table of the detailed constituents of the tea tree oil (see Appendix B).

This book is dedicated to my brother Alex and his wife Chiara, who in the early years of my interest and involvement with aromatherapy and herbalism provided both assistance and encouragement.

Introduction

Glancing through the contents of this book it would be easy to wonder how it is possible that one substance – tea tree oil – can be used to treat such a wide variety of complaints. On closer examination, however, the majority of the common ailments mentioned fall into three main categories: viral infections (such as chickenpox, measles or flu), fungal infections (such as athlete's foot, thrush or ringworm), and bacterial infections (such as infected cuts, spots or wounds). This is the unique strength of tea tree oil: it is effective against all three types of invasive organisms!

Natural remedies such as tea tree have enjoyed a great revival of interest in Europe and the US in recent years, as the general public have become increasingly disillusioned with aspects of the orthodox medical approach. The trend in modern Western medical practice has been to treat each disease or symptom with a specific, isolated chemical drug. While the scientific advances of the last century have in many ways brought significant benefits to the field of medicine, the drive towards specialization has also meant that the needs of the individual as a whole have tended to suffer. By concentrating on the physical manifestation of disease and its treatment, the emotional or psychological elements have been diminished and the human condition reduced by and large to the level of a chemical or molecular interaction.

In addition, though many of the newly developed drugs were found to target successfully the *symptoms* of disease, in the long term some of them also revealed detrimental side-effects. Such drawbacks include, for example, the addictive tendency of many prescribed sleeping pills and the gradual breakdown of the body's natural immunity to disease through the prolonged use of synthetically produced drugs such as antibiotics. Tea tree oil, in contrast, produces no side-effects in general, and boosts the immune system by supporting the body's own curative powers.

Over the last few years an increasing number of people have sought the help of 'alternative' or 'complementary' forms of healing, including herbal medicine/ phytotherapy and aromatherapy. What distinguishes these disciplines from the allopathic model? The main difference is that they take a 'holistic' approach, i.e. they assess the physical, emotional and spiritual needs of a patient as a whole. In this way, the overall harmony and sense of well-being which constitutes good health can be re-established. This is particularly relevant to our modern 20th-century life, where so many complaints – including stress and all its secondary effects – are often the result of underlying psychological issues. Based on an awareness of fundamental social problems, as well as a growing concern for the environment, there is now a strong trend towards a 'return to nature' – a more balanced lifestyle and a respect for the environment.

But the 'allopathic' and 'alternative' approaches need not be seen as working in opposition. Each has its own value; what is required today is an *integration* of modern science and traditional knowledge. In some Eastern countries such as China and India, traditional forms of medicine are employed alongside the newly adopted surgical skills and other modern techniques. In the West, too, these ancient healing methods are being reassessed. Such an exchange is very important, especially if we remember that many so-called 'alternative' methods are based on natural forms of healing which have been used for thousands of years within traditional cultures, whereas 'orthodox' medicine has hardly emerged from its infancy!

Herbal medicine, or phytotherapy, is one of the oldest traditional forms of healing. Plant-based medicines are also universal, for they were used by all ancient cultures – each developing its own individual system depending on its local flora. The Europeans and Native Americans, like every other indigenous race, once enjoyed a strong herbal tradition based on what grew around them. In Australia, for example, the Aborigine people were familiar with a number of aromatic plants which could be used as remedies, notably the eucalyptus (*Eucalyptus globulus*) and tea tree (*Melaleuca alternifolia*) – both plants rich in valuable essential oils.

The tea tree plant (*Melaleuca alternifolia*) produces one of the most medicinally active essential oils, which in recent years has gained increasing recognition from both alternative practitioners and within orthodox medical circles. This colourless or pale yellowy-green essential oil with its fresh, spicy-medicinal scent is now widely available and commonly known simply as 'tea tree' oil – although it is also sometimes referred to as 'ti-tree' or 'ti-trol'. It has gained an especially high profile in the context of 'aromatherapy' over the last few years – a modern 'alternative' or 'complementary' form of healing which has enjoyed a growing popularity since the late 1970s. Like herbal medicine, the practice known as 'aromatherapy' is also an ancient plant-based form of healing, but whereas medical herbalism utilizes the whole plant, aromatherapy uses only the essential oils from the plant – the aromatic aspect which gives each plant its scent.

Tea tree oil is an invaluable oil to the aromatherapist because of its numerous applications. It has superb antiseptic qualities and can be used simply and safely to treat a multitude of common complaints. Ease of use also makes it suitable for a wide range of first-aid applications, and as such it makes an invaluable addition to the household medicine cabinet or travel kit. Preparations using tea tree oil are also increasingly being used in a professional context in place of synthetic medications by more 'orthodox' practitioners, for it has been the subject of several intensive scientific investigations over the last few decades. Tea tree has been tested as a germicide (in Australia in 1980) in a solution of only 4 parts essential oil to 1000 parts water, with great success. According to one Australian doctor it will only be a matter of time before tea tree oil is recognized as 'the antiseptic of the future'. Tea tree need no longer be seen as something of a 'fad' – nor does it need to be restricted to the field of 'aromatherapy', for its applications and uses are more far reaching. Quite simply ...

> The basic message about tea tree is that here we have one of the most marvellous healing resources that nature has to offer ... [1]

Tea Tree's Medical and Historical Background

PART ONE

Native Folk Remedy of
the Australian Aborigines

TEA TREE OIL

The Narrow-leaved Paperbark Tea tree (*Melaleuca alternifolia*) is one member of an extensive botanical family, the Myrtaceae. All the plants belonging to this family are aromatic because they have glandular dots in their leaves which, when crushed, release essential oils of varying amounts and constituents.

Many plants in Australia (including Eucalyptus) belong to the Myrtaceae family, so it holds great prominence in the Australian flora. Like the Eucalyptus genus, of which there are hundreds of different sub-species, the *Melaleuca* and *Leptospermum* genera also form a large group which in Australia are known collectively as 'tea trees'. The fact that the same name is commonly used to describe a very diverse and widespread botanical group of plants indigenous to the region has naturally led to some confusion. This has been compounded by the fact that the essential oil derived from *Melaleuca alternifolia* has also been called 'ti-tree' oil, although 'ti' is the Maori name for an entirely different palm-like plant, the Cabbage tree (*Cordyline australis*).

The Narrow-leaved Paperback Tea tree is found only in Australia and is the smallest of the 'tea trees', not usually exceeding 20 ft/7 m in height. This spindly shrub with soft, bright green needle-like leaves and tiny yellow or cream 'bottle-brush' flowers thrives in swampy areas, being particularly abundant in the coastal wetlands of northern New South Wales and southern Queensland. The tea trees were formerly regarded as pests by immigrant dairy farmers because they made the land very difficult to clear. Having a very vigorous habit of growth, new shoots appeared very quickly after the trees were cut down, which made them virtually impossible to eradicate completely unless all the roots were dug out. It was only when the commercial value of tea tree itself became apparent in the early part of this century that this characteristic came to be appreciated rather than cursed!

The 'tea plant' was first mentioned in 1770, when Captain James Cook of the British Royal Navy landed on H.M.S. *Endeavour* at Botany Bay, on the southeast coast of Australia. During his exploration of this region (now New South Wales), as well as on his trip to New Zealand, he encountered thick groves of trees with aromatic leaves. A botanist with the expedition, Sir Joseph Banks, collected samples of the leaves gathered in New Zealand and brought them back to England for further study. An illustration of the shrub shows it to resemble Manuka (*Leptospermum scoparium*). Captain Cook called these 'tea plants' because their leaves, when boiled, produced a pleasant spicy and refreshing tea. He also used them for making home brewed beer:

> We at first made it – the beer – of a decoction of spruce leaves; but finding that this alone made the beer too astringent, we afterwards mixed with it an equal quantity of the tea plant (a name it obtained in my former voyage from our using it as tea then, as we also did

now) which partly destroyed the astringency of the other, and made the beer exceedingly palatable, and esteemed by everyone on board.[1]

The name 'tea tree' was apparently first coined by members of the First Fleet, as recorded by the surgeon of the expedition, General John White in his book *Journal of a Voyage to New South Wales* in 1790. He describes and illustrates a 'tea tree' that looks like another member of the *Leptospermum* group, possibly *L. attenuatum*, which was presumably used for brewing tea in the same way as Manuka or the more popular Sweet Sarsaparilla (*Smilax glycophylla*). By the early nineteenth century the name 'tea tree' was, however, widely used for members of the *Melaleuca* and *Leptospermum* group as a whole, and by 1820 one area of New South Wales was called 'Tea Tree Brush'.

The practice of making a beverage from the fragrant leaves most probably derived from its usage by the Bundjalung Aborigines who inhabited the area. The Aborigines were also familiar with the therapeutic properties of the 'tea tree' family, including *Melaleuca alternifolia*, and had used it as a traditional medicine for centuries.

> Aborigines used a number of tea trees in medicine. For coughs and colds, leaves were crushed and inhaled or soaked to make an infusion. Leaf washes were applied to pains, sores and burns.[2]

The crushed leaves, sometimes in combination with a warm mud pack, were also used to treat infections and a wide range of skin conditions. When, during the late 18th/early 19th century the white settlers arrived in Australia by their thousands, they naturally absorbed some of the native aboriginal practices. Eucalyptus, a well-known folk cure, became the basis of numerous remedies for many complaints throughout the Colony, while tea tree was used as an effective 'bush remedy' for all types of infection. The therapeutic properties of other indigenous plants such as sarsaparilla, maidenhair fern and myrtle were also gradually taken up by the early settlers. This was encouraged by Denis Considen, the first assistant surgeon to the Colony, who took great interest in the local flora with respect to its medical potential.

However, the lack of precise botanical or medical training on the part of most of the early explorers or settlers led to difficulties in the reliable assessment of the various species and the consequent acceptance of their benefits outside of Australia. Another problem stemmed from the general belief that it was only from those plants which were botanically closely related to known drug plants that new and effective medicines might be developed. In 1780, for example, John White – the Surgeon-General to the Colony – wrote highly of the properties of *Eucalyptus piperita* on account of:

> ... the very great resemblance between the essential oil drawn from its leaves and that obtained from the 'peppermint' (Mentha piperita) which grows in England.[3]

Indeed little serious attention was paid in Europe to the exact knowledge of the Aborigines, since most researchers regarded them simply as 'primitive' or 'uncivilized' beings whose chief interest lay in finding food. In contrast to many European herbs which had already enjoyed a long history of use, tea tree consequently only emerged in the West as a pharmacologically active agent during the 20th century — Australian tea tree oil being first mentioned in the British Pharmaceutical Codex of 1949.

Early Medical Research Reports

Tea tree is an oil which has received a great deal of attention at the hands of the scientific establishment during this century, despite its late arrival on the scene. This is important not only because the research results have finally begun to give tea tree credibility in orthodox medical circles, but also because it is an outstanding example of how folk lore and usage ascribed to a traditional remedy have been borne out and authenticated by scientific examination.

The first research project of this kind was carried out in 1923 by Dr A. R. Penfold, an Australian government chemist. He conducted a study of tea tree leaves and found that they contained an essential oil which exhibited antiseptic and bactericidal properties 13 times stronger than those of carbolic acid, the accepted standard of the time. When, in 1925, he announced his remarkable results before the Royal Society of New South Wales, he generated great enthusiasm among his medical colleagues and his 'discovery' was immediately put to the test. Over the next few years, tea tree oil was used experimentally in general practice as an antiseptic/bactericidal agent to treat a variety of complaints, and was found to be especially successful in the treatment of septic conditions, pus-filled infections, and dirty wounds. In 1930, an article entitled 'A New

Australian Germicide' appeared in *The Medical Journal of Australia* written by a Mr E. M. Humphrey, in which he stated that:

> The results obtained in a variety of conditions when it was first tried
> were most encouraging, a striking feature being that it dissolved pus
> and left the surfaces of infected wounds clean, so that its germicidal
> action became more effective without any apparent damage to the
> tissues. This was something new, as most effective germicides destroy
> tissue as well as bacteria.[1]

In addition, Humphrey noted that tea tree oil made an excellent antiseptic mouthwash, of particular benefit in dentistry and for infections of the nasopharynx. He also found that the oil had outstanding deodorant properties and that its disinfectant action on the thyroid bacilli was over 60 times more powerful than that of ordinary hand soap.

An Australian dentist, impressed by the research of Penfold and Humphrey, decided to try out tea tree in his own work:

> After trying [it] out in several tests, I felt confident that in Ti-trol
> [tea tree oil] and Melasol [a soluble form] we have an antiseptic
> which more nearly answers the ideal than any I have previously
> tested for our special work, and in general surgery it should be of
> even greater value.[2]

Over the next few years many studies were carried out into the various applications of tea tree oil which were reported in medical journals worldwide: first locally in *The Medical Journal of Australia, The Australian Journal of Dentistry* and *The Australian Journal of Pharmacy*; then, as its reputation spread abroad, in *The Journal of the National Medical Association* (US) and *The British Medical Journal*. In 1936 *The Medical Journal of Australia* reported that an aqueous suspension of the oil had successfully treated a severe case of diabetic gangrene. The special points of interest in this case were: unusual distribution of the gangrene; healing of the wound without any suppuration; reorganization of slough and necrosed bone under antiseptic treatment; avoidance of irritation of the wound when dressing; minimum of antiseptic applications.[3]

Other reports from all over the world confirmed tea tree's value for throat and mouth infections and gynaecological disorders as well as for many parasitic and fungal skin conditions. In 1937 it was also confirmed that the oil's antiseptic properties were further increased by 10–12 per cent in the presence of pus, blood and other matter!

By the end of the 1930s tea tree oil had gained the reputation of a natural 'miracle healer' – it was held in such high esteem that when the Second World War broke out it became standard issue in first-aid kits for Army and Naval units, especially those posted in tropical regions. Large quantities of the oil were also employed in munitions factories during the war, since by its incorporation (about 1 per cent) in machine 'cutting' oils, skin injuries, especially to the hands by metal filings, were greatly reduced.

But the extraordinary popularity which tea tree oil enjoyed during this period did not last ... with the growth of the synthetic drug industry it fell from favour as the medical establishment and the general public alike turned to man-made chemicals in search of new miracles!

Evidence Obtained from Later Clinical Studies

TEA TREE OIL

After the Second World War, as new synthetic germicides were developed, the medicinal value of pure tea tree oil was virtually forgotten – apart from in Australia where it remained a popular bush remedy. It was only during the 1960s, as a result of a growing awareness and concern regarding the hazardous side-effects of many of the newly manufactured drugs as well as their somewhat dubious financial and environmental implications, that natural remedies again began to attract widespread attention. Over the next few years a number of clinical studies were carried out into the effectiveness of tea tree oil for a wide range of conditions, although the most concrete evidence has emerged only recently. The following cases represent the chief 'milestones' of documented evidence:

1960

– Dr Henry Feinblatt reported in *The Journal of the National Medical Association* (US) that he had used pure tea tree oil twice a day to treat 25 cases of furunculosis (boils), with great success. After eight days, fifteen cases were cured completely, six boils were less than half their former size, three were substantially reduced ... only one needed incision. He concluded that tea tree oil 'encouraged more rapid healing without scarring than conservative treatment'.[1]

Early 1960s

– Dr E. F. Pena conducted a clinical study of 130 women suffering from various types of vaginal infection including trichomonal vaginitis, candida albicans (thrush) and cervicitis. Using a specially emulsified 40 per cent solution of pure oil of *Melaleuca alternifolia*, he obtained a clinical cure in all cases. His summary was as follows:

> Australian *Melaleuca alternifolia* oil in suitable dilutions was found to be highly effective in the treatment of trichomonal vaginitis, moniliasis, cervicitis and chronic endocervicitis ... Daily vaginal douches with 0.4 per cent of the oil in one quart of water proved safe and effective in treatment of the vaginal infections under consideration.[2]

1972

– Dr M. Walker conducted a study of various foot problems – athlete's foot, fungal infection, under-nail corns and callouses. Of 60 patients treated with pure tea tree oil, 58 were cured over a period which ranged from three weeks to six years. Of these 58 patients, excellent results occurred in 38 cases and fair effects in 20 cases.[3]

Early 1980s

– Prof. Paul Belaiche of the Phytotherapy Dept at the University of Paris carried out a series of studies using tea tree oil. One study involved 28 women suffering from the vaginal infection candida albicans (thrush). After 30 days of using tea tree oil (in the form of vaginal capsules inserted each evening) 21 cases were completely cured. The remaining seven were clinically but not biologically cured.

In a second study, a group of 26 women suffering from chronic cystitis were used in a double-blind test: 13 women were given 24 mg of tea tree oil daily (three doses of 8 mg before meals), while the other 13 were given a placebo tablet. After six months, seven out of the 13 in the first group were cured, compared to none in the second. Belaiche also used pure tea tree oil to treat a variety of fungal infections such as nailbed infections and paronychia as well as other skin disorders including acne and impetigo, with generally positive results.[4]

1983

– The Associated Foodstuff Laboratories of Australia conducted a series of skin sterilization trials using tea tree oil. By applying the essential oil to unwashed hands the bacteria count was reduced from 3,000 per 50 cm to 3 per 50 cm! The count on hands washed in distilled water, by comparison, was 2,000 per 50 cm.

1990

– A study involving 124 students was carried out by Prof. R. S. C. Barnetson at Sydney University to evaluate the efficacy and skin tolerance of a 5 per cent tea tree oil gel in the treatment of mild to moderate acne, in comparison with a 5 per cent benzoyl peroxide lotion (a widely used acne treatment). The results indicated that although the tea tree was slower to take effect, over the long term tea tree oil was equally efficient - with the added advantage that it caused fewer harsh side-effects. The researchers concluded that increased concentration of tea tree oil may even prove to be faster in its activity than the benzoyl peroxide lotion, and without causing any ill-effects.[5]

1991

– Dr Blackwell of the Department of Genito-urinary Medicine in Swansea (Wales) reported the case of a patient suffering from a vaginal infection who opted to treat herself using a tea tree oil vaginal pessary (200 gm in a vegetable oil base) rather than follow the standard pharmaceutical regimen (metronidazole in this case). After five days the infection had cleared up – showing that 'tea tree oil in the treatment of bacterial vaginosis may be a safe, non-toxic alternative to standard antibiotic treatment especially in pregnancy'.[6]

1991

– A more generalized study was carried out by A. Shemesh and W. L. Mayo at San Juan Capistrano, California over a six-month period during 1991. In this case, tea tree was used in the forms of oil, cream or lozenges to treat a variety of different conditions including acne, monilia of the mouth and throat, monilia rashes, non-specific dermatitis, eczema, oral canker sores, pustules, herpes simplex, fungus of the fingernails, and *Tinea cruris, pedis* and *barbae*. The test group consisted of 18 men, 30 women and 2 children; of all these patients only one (with eczema) was resistant to the treatment. All the other patients were cured or showed remarkable improvement in their presenting condition. Shemesh and Mayo concluded:

> Tea tree oil offers a natural, less expensive, effective alternative to currently used drugs for the described conditions in this study. It is safe, easily accessible and its side-effects profile is superior to most products currently prescribed for these medical problems.[7]

Production, Chemical Composition and Quality Control

TEA TREE OIL

Due to its fast-growing medical reputation, tea tree oil from *Melaleuca alternifolia* is now an expanding international industry. Whereas originally all the essential oil available was distilled from wild trees growing in one small region of New South Wales, it has now developed into a worldwide operation.

In the 1950s, there were just three field stills operating in the Bungawalbyn Valley – a swampy area where vast groves of the trees grew naturally. Since the trees grew in such inhospitable terrain, the harvesting was carried out on foot by individual bush-cutters, each one of whom carried only a supply of large hessian bags and a sharp knife. The trees were cut to within 2 m (7 ft) of the ground, and the leaves and branches were separated from the limbs. A good cutter could strip nearly one tonne of leaves in a day; these would then be carried directly to the still and emptied into large vats or pots. Using a wood-fired distillation unit, the essential oil was then extracted from the leaves using steam before being condensed and filtered. About one tonne of leaves was necessary to produce 6–10 kilos of essential oil – a yield of approximately 1 per cent.

It was only in the 1970s that the first tea tree farm was established in Bungawalbyn Creek with the aim of producing tea tree essential oil on a commercial scale. Even as late as 1988, however, most tea tree oil was still harvested and produced in the traditional manner.

Today, because of worldwide demand, the product relies increasingly on plantation production and sophisticated technology. Since 1988, several large plantations have been set up in a number of different areas such as Nambucca, Taree and Hornsby – a virgin crop is also being developed in California. The cultivation of tea trees has presented a new challenge, since on the first plots where the tea trees grew wild, replanting was unnecessary. In fact, far from damaging the trees, the regular cutting and pruning actually stimulated new growth, as is evident from the healthy trees in Bungawalbyn Creek which have been harvested regularly for over 60 years! The new growth, known as *ratoon*, takes only 18 months–2 years to reach a state of maturity, when it can be harvested again.

Since the cultivation of tea trees is a new kind of agriculture and there is still a great deal to be learned about the trees' optimum growing conditions. Factors which need to be assessed include how far apart the trees should be planted (to allow for mechanical harvesting), whether it is better to grow them from seed or propagate them by cuttings, and the exact chemical composition of the oil.

In its natural state, tea tree oil is an extremely complex chemical substance containing at least 48 organic compounds. The main constituents are terpenes, pinenes, cymones, terpineols, cineole, sesquiterpines and sesquiterpenine alcohols – however, it also contains four constituents that are rarely found elsewhere in nature: viridiflorine (approximately 1 per cent), B terpineol (0.24 per cent), L-terpineol (trace) and allyhexanoate (trace).[1] Variations in the constituents and properties of the essential oils produced from specially selected trees also need to be monitored closely. In 1948, Penfold, Morrison and McKern had already shown that the cineole content in a random sample of essential oils taken from 49 tea trees in the New South Wales region could vary between 6 per cent and 16 per cent, although the trees themselves were botanically indistinguishable. The proportion of cineole in tea tree oil has more recently been found to lie anywhere between 2 per cent and 65 per cent! The yield of oil has also been found to be lower in the winter months than in the summer.

Indeed, the standardization of tea tree oil has created some difficulty, since tea tree plants of identical botanical origin can produce essential oils of quite diverse composition – which consequently affects their healing potential. This is a pattern common to many aromatics – including thyme, lavender and marjoram – where the type and quality of an essential oil depends on factors such as altitude, seasonal changes and soil make-up.

When different essential oils can be produced from a single botanical species, grown under different circumstances, they are known as 'chemotypes'. These chemotypes are usually classified according to their main constituents, for example, tea tree is classified according to the amount of cineole (eucalyptol) and terpinen-4-ol that it contains.

Cineole has useful medicinal qualities, especially for the relief of respiratory complaints, but it is also an irritant of the mucous membranes and the skin. This means that tea tree oil containing large amounts of cineole is no good for using topically in the treatment of wounds, skin rashes, etc. The exclusive use of the low-cineole forms of tea tree oil for medical purposes has been highlighted in a series of research studies, notably by Penfold and Morrison (1946), Guenther (1950), and Lassak and McKarthy (1983). These factors were then used as a basis for standardization by the British Pharmaceutical Codex (1949) and the Standards Association of Australia (1967, 1985).

The Australian standard for *Melaleuca alternifolia* oil now requires that the terpinen-4-ol content of the oil should be greater than 30 per cent, and the cineole content less than 15 per cent. A top quality tea tree oil should, however, have a maximum cineole content of 5 per cent and a minimum terpinen-4-ol content of 35–40 per cent. As the demand for tea tree has increased, the essential oil has also been increasingly subjected to adulteration, usually with cineole – the main constituent of eucalyptus oil which gives the eucalyptus oil its characteristic camphor-like scent. A tea tree oil which has been tampered with in this way can be identified by its sweetish, light aroma and its strong camphor-like note. Nowadays the different constituents of tea tree are measured using a gas chromatograph – where the presence and position of each peak on the graph shows the amount of each component. The balance of the main constituents in a fresh, high quality tea tree oil should be approximately as follows:

Alpha-pinene	2.5 per cent
Alpha-terpinene	9.1 per cent

Para-cymene	3.9 per cent
1,8-cineole	4.3 per cent
Gamma-terpinene	24.6 per cent
Alpha-terpineol	2.3 per cent
Terpinen-4-ol	42.1 per cent
Terpinolene	4.1 per cent

It is interesting to note that none of these substances is especially effective alone. It is only in combination that these substances demonstrate their maximum healing power – which is known as a 'synergy'. This is a quality common to many essential oils, where the unique balance of constituents, including the trace elements, contributes to the overall effectiveness of the remedy. This factor also helps to account for why synthetically produced products, or 'nature-identical' oils, cannot match properties exhibited by the naturally derived original, since it is very difficult to mimic the complex and diverse blend of components found in nature.

Detailed research into the exact properties of different types of tea tree oils is being carried out at present to ascertain and identify the most suitable composition for particular medicinal applications. As the tea tree industry becomes more sophisticated it is more than likely that specific oils will be prepared for each condition – for example, the optimum composition for combating a fungal condition may not be the same as that for a bactericidal infection. With regard to candida, for example, it has been found that there is a general decline in activity as the levels of the following components decrease: alpha-terpinene, gamma-terpinene, terpinolene, terpinen-4-ol; and as the level of the following compounds increase; cineole, limonene, alpha-terpineol.

NOTE

See Appendix B for a more detailed survey of the constituents of tea tree oil.

A Summary of the Properties and Applications of Tea Tree Oil

TEA TREE OIL

Due to its unique composition, tea tree oil displays a number of remarkable properties making it very effective for a wide range of complaints. Foremost among these properties, and what makes tea tree oil outstanding in comparison to other remedies, is that it is active against all three varieties of infectious organisms: bacteria, fungi and viruses. Independent microbiological testing has confirmed the effectiveness of tea tree oil against a wide range of micro-organisms, notably:

> **Gram Positive bacteria:** *Staphyloccus aureus, Staphyloccus epidermidis, Staphyloccus pneumoniae, Staphyloccus faecalis, Staphyloccus pyrogenes, Staphyloccus agalactiae, Propioni-bacterium acnes, Beta haemolytic streptococcus*
>
> **Gram Negative bacteria:** *Escherichia coli, Klebsiella pneumoniac, Citrobacter spp., Shigella sonnei, Proteus mirabilis, Legionella spp., Pseudomonas aeruginosa*
>
> **Fungi:** *Trichophyton mentagrophytes, Trichophyton rubrum, Aspergillus niger, Aspergillus flavus, Candida albicans, Microsporum canis, Microsporum gypseum, Thermoactinomycetes vulgaris.*

Tea tree's effectiveness in fighting infection is further backed up by its ability to stimulate the immune system – this means that if the body is threatened by any of these organisms, tea tree increases the body's own ability to protect itself and to respond appropriately. Tea tree oil's main areas of activity may therefore be summarized as: antiseptic/bactericidal, anti-fungal, anti-viral, and immuno-stimulant. Its secondary properties are also looked at in detail below.

Antiseptic/Bactericidal

This property of tea tree makes it excellent for first aid – i.e. the treatment of cuts, burns, insect bites, infected splinters and all kinds of wounds (especially those which are dirty or contain pus). As an antiseptic, tea tree is also very valuable for general skin care, notably for spots, acne, blackheads, etc. As a general disinfectant it is especially useful for respiratory or genito-urinary tract infections such as bronchitis and sinusitis or cystitis.

Anti-fungal

Tea tree oil's excellent fungicidal qualities make it a very effective treatment for a wide range of common complaints including ringworm, athlete's foot and thrush (candida). It has also been used with great success to combat fungal diseases affecting animals, fish and plants.

Anti-viral

Viruses are the invading organisms responsible for most epidemic illnesses. As a powerful anti-viral agent, tea tree is effective in fighting many common infectious diseases such as measles, chickenpox, flu, colds and shingles as well as other viral complaints such as cold sores, veruccae and warts.

Immuno-stimulant

In this context, tea tree is principally of great value as a *preventative* remedy – to help the body fight off all kinds of infection. This is especially important if the body is already in a weakened condition brought on by either stress, illness or the use of anti-biotics or other drugs which have lowered the body's natural resistance levels. Tea tree has been found to be especially helpful for those who need to have their strength built up, such as before a surgical operation or for those suffering from chronic or long-standing debilitating illnesses such as glandular fever or hepatitis. Its possible application to AIDS is also currently being researched.

Secondary Properties

In addition, tea tree oil has several secondary properties or actions:

Its value as an external remedy for complaints affecting the skin (including cuts, burns and bruises) is furthered by its **anti-inflammatory**, **analgesic** (pain-killing) and **cicatrizant** (wound-healing) qualities.

It is also a powerful **parasiticide** and **insecticide** – effective against many types of infestations including lice, scabies, mosquitoes, etc.

It has a **diaphoretic** effect – that is, it promotes sweating – which again enhances the body's own natural preventative response when threatened by infection.

Finally, tea tree exhibits **expectorant** and **balsamic** characteristics, which are especially beneficial in the case of throat or chest infections, having a generally soothing and clearing (mucus-expelling) effect on the entire respiratory tract.

Methods of Use, Safety Data and Storage Precautions

TEA TREE OIL

Methods of Use

Tea Tree in the Bath

Add 8–10 drops to the bath water once the bath is full, then relax in the water for at least 10 minutes.

For bathing the feet or hands, add 6–8 drops of tea tree oil to a bowl or shallow bath of warm water and soak for 5–10 minutes.

As a Compress/Poultice

A simple disinfectant compress can be made by dipping a flannel (face-cloth) or piece of cotton wool (cotton ball) in a bowl of water (either steaming hot or ice cold, as required) to which has been added 3–5 drops of tea tree oil. A poultice (to draw pus from abscesses or infected splinters, etc.) can be made by adding a few drops of tea tree to a clay or kaolin base, and mixing well.

Direct/Neat Application

Use the oil direct from the bottle – dabbing with the fingertips or using a cotton bud (cotton swab) – to treat cuts, burns, cold sores, etc.

A few people find neat tea tree irritating to the skin – if irritation does occur, bathe with cold water and in future use in low dilutions only (or avoid altogether).

Gargling and Dental Care

For the treatment of mouth ulcers, sore throats, bad breath or other mouth and gum infections, add 5–10 drops of tea tree oil to a glass of warm water, mix well, then rinse the mouth and/or gargle.

Inhalation

Use up to 8 drops on a tissue or handkerchief for inhalation throughout the day (or onto a pillow for night use). For respiratory complaints, make a steam inhalation by adding about 5 drops of tea tree to a bowl of steaming water. Cover your head with a towel and breathe deeply for about 5–10 minutes with your eyes closed. Steam inhalation also acts as a kind of facial 'sauna' – used in this way tea tree can help unblock the pores and clear the skin of acne, spots and blackheads.

Massage

Before being applied to the skin for massage purposes, tea tree (like other essential oils) should always be mixed with a light vegetable oil carrier or base such as sweet almond oil, jojoba or grapeseed – although sunflower or soya oil would also suffice. Jojoba oil, being a liquid wax, does not go rancid – otherwise a little wheatgerm oil should be added to the blend to prolong its shelf life. The dilution should be in the region of 2–3 per cent – though sometimes 5 per cent may be used for a concentrated effect, as in the case of local muscular pain, for example.

A rough guideline is to say that 20 drops of tea tree oil is equivalent to one millilitre, so an easy way of calculating the proportions for general use is to measure the carrier oil in millilitres, then add about half the number of drops of tea tree oil to give a 2.5 per cent dilution:

100 ml base oil	50 drops essential oil
50 ml base oil	25 drops essential oil
1 tbsp (approx. 15 ml) base oil	7–8 drops essential oil
1 tsp (approx. 5 ml) base oil	2–3 drops essential oil

Shampoo and Hair Care

A 3–4 per cent dilution of tea tree is common in commercial tea tree shampoos and soaps. Otherwise buy a good, neutral pH value shampoo and add your own tea tree to it: to a 100-ml bottle add about 60 drops. This disinfects the hair and is good for the prevention and/or cure of dandruff and lice. An alcohol-based scalp rub can be made by adding 5 ml of tea tree to 100 ml of vodka – this can be used to rid the hair of fleas and lice (but note that alcohol should not be used on irritated skin).

Sitz Bath/Douche

For vaginal and genito-urinary infections, add a few drops of tea tree oil to a shallow bath or bowl of warm water and bathe the affected area.

Skin Treatments: Creams, Gels, Lotions, Masks and Oils

The proportions used for mixing skin creams, gels, masks and oils are the same as those for massage purposes – see p. 29.

A light water-based lotion can be made up using 100 ml distilled water and 25 drops of tea tree oil – shake well before use. For some conditions (such as cold sores and athlete's foot) it is better to use an alcohol-based lotion because it is more drying. This can be made by adding 6 drops of tea tree to 5 ml of neat vodka. This mixture can be further diluted in a litre of boiled/cooled water for treating cuts and sores, such as those caused by chickenpox.

Vaporization

There are many vaporizing methods available now – you may use an essential oil burner, an electric diffuser, or you can simply put a few drops of tea tree oil in a small bowl of hot water placed on a radiator or any other source of heat. This method is particularly useful for disinfecting a sick room and preventing the spread of contagious illness. Tea tree may also be used to repel insects in this manner.

Other Measures

Many common conditions benefit from combining aromatherapy with other approaches such as herbal medicine, acupuncture, counselling, dietary changes and exercise. Essential oils and allopathic medicines can also complement one another – check with a qualified herbalist or aromatherapy practitioner for further advice.

Safety Data

Tea tree is generally non-toxic, non-irritating and non-sensitizing. It does not destroy healthy skin tissue, only pathogens. Sensitization to tea tree oil has occasionally been encountered; extremely sensitive skin may require a dilution of the pure oil or may need to avoid it altogether. In one case reported in 1992 a woman with atopic dermatitis was treated with neat tea tree oil applied directly to the skin.[1] When the condition worsened, oral ingestion was prescribed, which only exacerbated the problem. On investigation, cineole was found to be the allergen. In another case a boy with athlete's foot was treated with tea tree oil which aggravated the condition further.[2] Later it was discovered that he had had an allergic reaction to tea tree oil – again possibly due to its cineole content.

Before using tea tree oil for the first time it is best to carry out a 'patch test' – simply apply a few drops of tea tree to the back of the wrist and leave for 1 hour. If any irritation occurs, bathe with cold water and use tea tree only in dilution or avoid it altogether in the future.

Babies, young children and pregnant women should take special care using all essential oils, because of their concentration. Despite tea tree's low toxicity level, it is advisable not to use it neat for the treatment of children under 18 months of age – and always dilute for use during pregnancy to half the usual concentration.

Pet owners are also advised not to use full-strength tea tree oil on small animals.

In common with all essential oils, tea tree should not be taken internally (unless under strict medical supervision); it is sufficiently toxic to cause concern if quantities such as 5 ml or more are ingested by young children.

Storage

For storage purposes tea tree oil should be treated like a citrus oil as it is prone to oxidation upon exposure to air. When this occurs, the Gamma-terpinene content decreases and the para-cymene content increases. The terpinen-4-ol content, the active microbiol constituent, is also reduced but not as drastically. This means that if the oil is not stored correctly it becomes less and less bacteri-cidal. It should be kept in an airtight dark-glass container, away from light and heat and well out of the reach of children or pets. The pure oil will also dissolve certain plastics, so good care should be taken regarding any substances the neat oil comes into contact with.

IT IS VERY IMPORTANT TO OBTAIN PURE TEA TREE OIL FROM A REPUTABLE SOURCE TO ENSURE A SAFE AND EFFECTIVE THERAPEUTIC RESULT!

A–Z of Health Care Applications

Applications

PART TWO

Acne (and Spots)

This unsightly skin condition is caused by an overactivity of the sebaceous glands, and is especially common during adolescence, the menopause and at times of hormonal upheaval, such as before or during menstruation.

A very greasy, congested skin results in a rough surface texture, enlarged pores, spots, pimples and blackheads. The condition can be exacerbated further by a poor diet, too little exercise, lack of hygiene, stress and other emotional factors. Scrupulous attention to hygiene prevents the condition spreading – wash gently with an unscented pH-balanced soap, or a tea tree soap. The effectiveness and success of tea tree in combating acne has been well researched by recent clinical studies (see pages 15 and 16).

- Apply neat tea tree oil to individual spots night and morning using a cotton bud (cotton swab).
- Make up a lotion using 100 ml distilled water and 25 drops of tea tree oil. Shake well before use and bathe the face (and other affected areas) night and morning.
- Make up a 5 per cent non-oily cream or gel (see pages 29–30), or use a commercial tea tree ointment to apply as a cleansing/moisturizing ointment.

- Add 8–10 drops of tea tree oil to the bath water – this also acts as a facial steam (see page 27, Methods of Use).
- Have a facial sauna 3 or 4 times a week using 3–5 drops of tea tree (see page 28, Methods of Use).
- Other oils of benefit: lavender, bergamot, geranium.

Arthritis (and Gout)

There are several different kinds of arthritis – but all signify the body's inability to eliminate toxic waste efficiently. This causes excess uric acid to be deposited as crystals in the joint spaces. The two most common forms are *rheumatoid arthritis*, which can affect all age groups, and *osteoarthritis*, which usually occurs in the elderly. Both are forms of joint distress which can result in pain, inflammation and sometimes deformity.

Gout usually affects the joints of the toes, but also sometimes the fingers.

Stress, emotional conflict, lack of exercise and a poor diet all contribute to these conditions. Aromatic baths and massage can help eliminate the toxic waste, as well as provide relief from pain.

- Make a massage oil by mixing 30 drops of tea tree oil with 50 ml of a vegetable carrier oil. Apply twice daily.
- Add 8–10 drops of tea tree oil to the bath water for pain relief.
- To ease inflammation, apply a cold compress using clay (or a flannel or face-cloth) to which has been added a few drops of tea tree oil.

- *Note:* There are several other oils which are of great benefit in arthritis: *for detoxifying* – cypress, fennel, juniper and lemon; *for pain relief* – chamomile, lavender and marjoram; and *for stimulating greater mobility* – pine, rosemary and ginger.

Athlete's foot

Athlete's foot is a fungal infection caused by *Tinea pedis*, commonly characterized by red, soggy or flaky skin and itching between the toes. Sometimes the soles and heels become covered in white scaly skin – it may also affect the fingers or nails.

The affected skin usually becomes cracked and painful, and in such cases the feet should be allowed to 'breathe' whenever possible. Athlete's foot is often picked up in sports' changing rooms and schools as it is highly contagious. Tea tree has been found to be very effective in treating this condition.

- Wash and dry the feet thoroughly, then apply neat tea tree to the affected areas. Continue to apply 2 or 3 times daily until the condition has cleared up.
- Soaking the feet for 5–10 minutes a day in a tea tree foot bath (5–10 drops in a bowl of warm water) is also beneficial.
- In addition, add 8–10 drops of tea tree to the bath as a precautionary measure.

See also **Tinea**

Balanitis

Balanitis is an irritating condition affecting the end of the penis; it is caused by the fungal infection *Candida albicans*. It is usually contracted from sexual contact with a woman suffering from thrush, a vaginal infection caused by the same organism. With balanitis or thrush it is important that both male and female sexual partners are treated simultaneously before renewing sexual relations, to avoid re-infection.

- Balanitis may be treated by washing the area carefully with a 1 per cent solution of tea tree in distilled water (shaken well) applied 4 times a day.

See also **Candida** and **Thrush**

Barber's Rash

Barber's rash, sometimes known as 'shaving rash', is caused by the fungal infection *Tinea barbae*. It is characterized by a mass of small red pimples on the face and neck – the skin is also often flaky and sore. The condition is aggravated by shaving and can be compounded by acne.

- Make up a soothing lotion using 3–5 drops of tea tree in 1 tsp water-based gel and apply morning and night. (Avoid using harsh soaps or commercial after-shaves).

See also **Tinea**

Boil (Furuncle)/Abscess

A boil or abscess is a localized painful swelling and inflammation of the skin, due to an infection of a sebaceous gland.

Boils usually appear when the body is run-down or stressed, at times of hormonal upheavel or as the result of a blood disorder. Whatever the cause, the presence of a boil or abscess indicates that the system is in need of purification. Avoid stimulants, eat lots of fresh fruit and vegetables and drink plenty of water or herb teas (especially those which purify the blood).

Medical research has affirmed that tea tree is an excellent treatment for boils and abscesses because it penetrates through the skin to combat the infection and disperses the pus without making it necessary to break the skin (for further evidence see page 12).

- Never wait for the boil or abscess to burst – treat as soon as it begins to appear by dabbing with neat tea tree oil. Repeat 2 or 3 times a day.
- If the boil/abscess has already formed, apply a warm poultice of clay containing 3–4 drops of tea tree oil. Leave for half an hour to draw the liquid/pus, then bathe gently with water. Alternatively, apply a warm flannel (face-cloth) which has been soaked in a tea tree solution, then dab the boil with neat tea tree oil. Repeat 2 or 3 times a day.

- If the boil/abscess is severe, cover with a gauze soaked in tea tree oil for 12 hours. If there is still no improvement, seek medical advice.
- Add 8–10 drops of tea tree oil to the bath water as a general disinfectant measure.
- Other oils of benefit: bergamot, chamomile, lavender.

Bites/Stings

– *see* **Insect Bites**

Bronchitis

Bronchitis indicates an inflammation of the bronchial tubes, accompanied by coughing and mucus congestion. Acute bronchitis usually starts with a cold or sore throat which then develops into a fever that lasts a few days. Chronic bronchitis is a long-term condition, without fever, which is aggravated by smoking, a damp climate, air pollution and poor nutrition (especially too many dairy products).

Tea tree can be of great benefit by helping to combat the infection, reduce fever, ease coughing and expel mucus. It can also help to reinforce the body's immune mechanism and prevent the infection from spreading.

NOTE

Bronchitis can lead to complications, especially in the very young and elderly – professional help should be sought immediately if the condition deteriorates.

- At the onset, regular steam inhalations will help to prevent the infection from developing and help to soothe coughing – add 5 drops of tea tree to a bowl of steaming hot water and inhale for 5–10 minutes.

- Hot baths with 8–10 drops of tea tree added encourage sweating, the body's natural response to infection – it also has a similar effect to steam inhalation. When feverish, especially if the temperature is high, keep the bath water cool.

- Massage the chest, back and throat with a 2.5 per cent blend of tea tree in a light base oil or cream – 3 drops to 1 tsp of cream or base oil.

- Use a vaporizer in the home, especially in the bedroom at night. A few drops of pure tea tree oil can also be put on a tissue or handkerchief for inhalation throughout the day.

- Other oils of benefit: eucalyptus, lavender.

See also **Colds, Coughs, Fever, Flu, Sinusitis, Sore Throat**

Bruises/Bumps

A bruise indicates that the tissue is damaged beneath the skin's surface as a result of a bump or pressure to that area. Applying tea tree oil reduces inflammation, heals cell tissues and speeds up the healing process.

Suppurating bruise of shin which appeared to be progressing to a condition of periostitis, checked in 24 hours using solution diluted 1 to 40 as a compress. Condition cured in one week by continuing this treatment.[1]

- Apply a cold compress to ease inflammation, then dab a drop or two of neat tea tree oil onto the affected area.
- Lavender essential oil and arnica ointment are also very useful bruise remedies.

Burns

Burns can be caused by dry heat or moist heat (scalds), and are often very painful. Minor burns respond extremely well to treatment with essential oils as they reduce the pain, prevent blistering or infection and promote healing.

NOTE

Severe burns, especially if accompanied by shock, require immediate medical attention.

Tea tree oil is increasingly employed in burn treatment products in Australia.

Apart from the rapid healing and absence of infection I have observed, one of the great benefits has been relief of pain with the initial application.[2]

- Immediately put the affected area under the cold tap for 5 minutes, then apply neat tea tree oil to the site of the burn. Continue to apply neat at least 3 times a day until the skin has healed.
- Alternatively, apply a water-based gel to which 5–10 per cent tea tree oil has been added.
- Other measures: lavender essential oil is also a very effective burn remedy when used in the same manner.

Candida

Candida, also known as *candidiasis* or *moniliasis*, can manifest in several forms. It is caused by the yeast-like fungal infection *Candida albicans* and thrives in moist, warm parts of the body including the mouth (*candidiasis*), beneath the breasts, on the penis (*balanitis*) and between the folds of the buttocks (the latter often occurring in babies as a type of nappy rash). In its most common form, however, (usually called 'thrush') it affects the vagina causing severe itching and a milky-white discharge.

For methods of treatment see **Balanitis, Mouth and Gum Infections, Nappy (Diaper) Rash, Thrush**

Carbuncles

A carbuncle is a collection of boils caused by *staphyloccus aureaus* – characterized by a painful node and covered with tight red skin that later becomes thick and discharges pus. Carbuncles are commonly found on the upper back, nape of the neck or the buttocks.

- Keep the area clean and apply neat tea tree oil to the site of the problem 3 times a day.
- Add 8–10 drops of tea tree to the bath water as a disinfectant measure.
- Lavender oil is also an effective remedy, used alone or in combination with tea tree.

Chickenpox

Chickenpox is a highly contagious viral infection – common during childhood – which is caused by herpes zoster, the same virus which is responsible for shingles (**zona**). A fever develops and itchy spots appear in crops; these spots progress to blisters and then to crusts.

Tea tree is very effective for chickenpox due to its anti-viral, immunostimulant, analgesic (pain-killing) and diaphoretic (sweat-promoting) properties. It also soothes itching and promotes healing of the spots – thus helping to prevent possible infection or scarring due to scratching. In one recorded case, an 11-month-old baby with a severe attack of chickenpox was bathed using 2 drops of tea tree oil and 1 drop of German chamomile in the water, and showed improvement within an hour. After two more baths, she slept soundly for most of the night.

> By morning, most of the blisters were 50 per cent smaller, and all those which erupted from this time onwards remained small. I bathed her twice a day with ti-tree until all the scabs had fallen off, and she

now has less scarring than Emma or Michael, despite the severity of the attack.[3]

In adults chickenpox can be more dangerous, as it is accompanied by a high temperature and pain. Another case history records the progress of a man suffering from chickenpox whose body (but not the skin on his face) was treated with an alcohol solution using tea tree as a dabbing lotion. He also gained great relief by bathing 3 times a day in a bath to which a blend of tea tree, lavender and chamomile had been added:

> The most interesting point to note in connection with the action of ti-tree, is that the very heavy crop of spots on his body cleared much faster than those on his face, many of them without reaching their full size, while most of the spots on his face developed into large blisters and scabbed over in the manner characteristic of chickenpox.[4]

- Use tea tree in vaporizers throughout the duration of the illness.
- Soak frequently using a blend of tea tree, lavender and chamomile in tepid water for 10–15 minutes at a time, every few hours if possible. For babies add 2 drops of tea tree and 1 drop of chamomile (or lavender) dissolved in 1 tsp of alcohol in the bath; for children add 3 drops of tea tree and 2 drops of chamomile (or lavender) dissolved in 1 tsp alcohol; for adults add 5 drops tea tree and 5 drops of chamomile (or lavender) dissolved in 1 tsp alcohol.

- Dissolve 25 (15 for children) drops of tea tree and 10 (5 for children) drops each of lavender and chamomile in one dessert-spoon of alcohol, then mix with 50 ml rosewater and 50 ml witch-hazel. Shake well before using – apply frequently to spots using a cotton wool or gauze pad.

  Note: this treatment is not suitable for young babies.
- Other measures: a handful of colloidal oatmeal (available from most chemists) may also be added to the bath water to soothe itching and encourage healing.

Chilblains

Chilblains are small, painful reddish-blue swellings which are sometimes itchy. They occur mostly on the toes or fingertips, usually as a result of poor circulation or cold. Vitamin and mineral deficiency can also contribute to the problem. Exercise and warm clothing are important preventative measures.

- Apply neat tea tree (or lemon juice) to the chilblain.
- A regular stimulating massage treatment is beneficial. Local blood circulation can be improved by massaging the feet or affected area with 2 drops each of tea tree and black pepper in 1 tsp carrier oil.

Colds

There are at least 30 different strains of the virus which can cause the common cold or, in medical terms, *coryza*. This highly contagious infection affects the upper respiratory tract. The symptoms are well known: sore throat, coughing, feverishness, aching limbs, sneezing, fatigue and catarrh.

Tea tree oil can do much to reduce the duration or severity of the illness and help to prevent secondary infections (such as bronchitis, sinusitis or ear infections) from arising. In addition, tea tree can often prevent the cold from developing at all if it is used at the onset, due to its powerful anti-viral and immuno-stimulant qualities.

- Use tea tree in vaporizers throughout the duration of the illness, but especially at the onset of the cold – this may prevent it from developing at all. In addition, add a few drops to a handkerchief for inhalation throughout the day, and to the pillow for night use.
- Take a daily hot bath adding 8–10 drops of tea tree to the water – this soothes aching limbs and also acts as a kind of steam inhalation.
- For a sore throat, add 5–10 drops of tea tree to a glass of warm water, mix well and gargle. Repeat 2 or 3 times a day at least.
- For a cough, make up a concentrated chest rub by mixing 5 drops of tea tree with 5 drops of marjoram (or benzoin) in 1 dessertspoon of carrier oil and apply to the chest and upper back. Repeat at least twice a day.

- As a steam inhalation, add 5–6 drops of tea tree oil to a bowl of steaming water, cover your head with a towel and breathe deeply for 5–10 minutes with your eyes closed ... very hot steam is in itself a hostile environment for viruses. Repeat at least twice a day.
- Other measures: take a course of garlic capsules and vitamin C tablets. Lavender, marjoram or chamomile oil can also be used in baths to soothe aching limbs and to encourage restful sleep.

See also **Coughs, Fever, Flu, Sinusitis, Sore Throat**

Cold Sores

A cold sore is a blister-like sore, usually found on the lips or face, caused by the virus *herpes simplex I*. The condition is infectious and can be spread to other parts of the body or to other people quite readily.

Some people are particularly prone to cold sores, especially when they are run down or have suffered exposure to cold winds or hot sunshine.

Tea tree has been found to be a very effective remedy for cold sores, especially if they are treated early on. The pure oil was used successfully to combat herpes simplex in the clinical study carried out by Shemesh and Mayo in 1991 (see pages 15–16) – several case histories also bear witness to its effectiveness in treating this stubborn virus:

> I have been suffering from cold sores for years, and they get quite bad at times to the point of leaving scar tissue on my face. My last

bout with this problem was much better, thanks to your tea tree oil. In fact, as I felt it coming on, I started using the tea tree oil and it never developed into a sore.[5]

- Use neat tea tree oil to dab the sore spot as soon as it begins to develop – if it is treated early enough it can stop the cold sore from developing altogether. Repeat frequently over a period of several days, or until the condition has cleared.
- Add 6 drops of tea tree oil to 1 tsp alcohol (such as vodka) – this alcohol-based lotion may be used in place of pure tea tree oil during the initial stages of treatment if the skin is not broken, otherwise it can cause a stinging sensation.
- Other measures: take vitamin C tablets; lavender and bergamot (bergapten-free) oil are also beneficial for treating cold sores when applied in the same manner as tea tree.

Corns

A corn or clavus is an area of hard thickened skin on or between the toes. It can form an inverted pyramid which presses into the deeper layers of skin, causing pain. In 1972, Dr Walker (see page 13) conducted a clinical study in which he used pure tea tree oil to treat a variety of foot problems including callouses and corns beneath the nails, with good results.

- Apply pure tea tree oil to the area using the tip of a finger or a cotton bud (cotton swab) and cover with a plaster (adhesive bandage). Repeat on a daily basis – it may take several weeks to see any results, but it is effective in the long run.

Coughs

Coughing is a natural reflex action aimed at clearing an obstruction or irritation from the respiratory tract. A cough can be dry and unproductive or it can be accompanied by a mucus discharge, especially when it occurs in association with a cold, flu or bronchitis. Tea tree oil, due to its powerful anti-viral, bactericidal, expectorant and balsamic properties, is a valuable remedy for coughs if there is any infection or inflammation involved.

- Add 5–6 drops of tea tree oil to a bowl of steaming water, cover your head with towel and breathe deeply for 5–10 minutes with your eyes closed. Repeat at least twice a day.
- Make up a concentrated chest rub by mixing 5 drops of tea tree with 5 drops of marjoram (or benzoin) in 1 dessertspoon of carrier oil and apply to the chest and upper back. Repeat at least twice a day.
- Use tea tree in vaporizers throughout the duration of the illness.
- Other measures: keep warm and protect the neck and throat region by wearing a scarf; eucalyptus sandalwood, pine, benzoin and thyme oil are also beneficial for coughs when used in a similar manner to tea tree oil.

See also **Bronchitis, Colds, Fever, Flu, Sinusitis, Sore Throat**

Cracked Skin

Dry, cracked skin on the feet and hands is a common problem, especially during the winter months. In severe cases it can be painful, especially in association with frostbite or skin complaints such as psoriasis.

- Mix 3 drops of tea tree with 1 tsp wheatgerm oil (or a thick moisturizing cream) and massage well into the affected area night and morning. Continue until the condition improves.
- Other measures; benzoin, lavender, myrrh and patchouli are also useful essential oils for cracked skin when used individually or in combination and applied in a similar fashion to tea tree oil.

Cradle Cap

This unsightly scalp condition is a form of dermatitis which affects very young babies, especially the newborn. A thick, yellowish crust develops on the scalp and there is often scaling behind the ears.

- Mix fresh for each treatment 5 drops of tea tree oil with 1 dessertspoon of slightly warmed olive oil – rub gently into the scalp. Leave for 5–10 minutes then wash out using tea tree shampoo (the scalp may remain slightly oily after the treatment). Take care to avoid the eyes while rinsing. Repeat daily initially, then continue using tea tree shampoo as part of the baby's normal routine to prevent a recurrence.

- ■ Lavender oil is also useful for cradle cap when used in the same manner as tea tree.

See also **Dermatitis/Eczema**

Cuts/Wounds

Small cuts and scratches are some of the most common household injuries, especially where young children are concerned. Tea tree is an ideal first-aid remedy for all sorts of minor skin abrasions due to its excellent antiseptic and wound-healing properties. It is so gentle that it does not sting the exposed raw skin, and it acts as a mild anaesthetic and encourages a rich flow of blood to the damaged area. In addition, tea tree oil has been found actually to work better in the presence of dirt or pus! (See E. M. Humphrey's research during the 1930s – page 9).

> A medical man in Evanston, Illinois [US] reports the successful treatment of a nasty head wound which, because of the hair, was disinclined to heal; Ti-trol [tea tree oil] effected a quick and healthy healing.[6]

- Clean the area thoroughly with water, then dab on a few drops of pure tea tree oil. Apply a plaster (adhesive bandage) if required. Continue to apply the tea tree oil neat, several times a day until the skin has healed.
- Other measures: pure lavender oil can be used as an alternative.

Cystitis/Urethritis

Cystitis is a bacterial infection of the bladder, more common among women than men. It is characterized by a frequent need to urinate, a painful burning sensation while passing water (which is often cloudy) and sometimes feverishness. Many attacks of cystitis start as urethritis – an infection of the urethra.

During the 1980s, Dr Paul Belaiche used tea tree oil experimentally to treat chronic cystitis with considerable success (see page 14). He concluded:

> From this first clinical approach it is apparent that the essential oil of *Melaleuca alternifolia* is effectively efficient for the treatment of chronic *colibacilli* cystitis. The absence of toxicity, the low level of irritation on the mucous membrane, its perfect general tolerance, and its high germicidal power ... has convinced us that we are in possession of a major new antiseptic essential oil for aromatherapy.[7]

Although Dr Belaiche's study (and other more recent cases) employed tea tree capsules taken internally as part of the treatment, the following types of external applications can be very effective in themselves, especially if undertaken immediately at the very first signs of irritation.

NOTE

Do not take tea tree internally without medical supervision; if symptoms do not improve within a few days, or if there is blood or pus in the urine, seek professional help immediately.

- Make up a solution using 10 drops of tea tree oil in half a litre of cooled boiled water. Using a piece of soaked cotton wool (a cotton ball), swab the opening of the urethra frequently (if possible, after each time you pass water).
- Add 8–10 drops to the bath water – it is beneficial to bathe frequently using bactericidal oils as a general disinfectant and preventative measure.
- Make up a massage oil using 3 drops of tea tree oil in 1 tsp light carrier oil (such as jojoba or grapeseed) and rub gently into the lower abdomen and back. Repeat at least twice daily.
- Other measures: drink plenty of water or herbal teas; avoid tight fitting clothes and nylon underwear; take a course of garlic capsules; bergamot, lavender, chamomile and sandalwood essential oils are also of benefit when used in a similar fashion to tea tree, or in combination with tea tree oil.

Dandruff

This common yet embarrassing problem is caused by *Candida albicans* – a fungus (also known as a yeast infection) which affects the scalp. The condition can be further aggravated by overactive sebaceous glands, excessive use of chemical hair preparations, a poor diet and stress.

Tea tree oil can do much to clear up this problem while at the same time improving the overall condition and health of the hair. In the words of one Australian doctor:

> Another condition for which I prescribe tea tree a lot is dandruff – a lot of people ... have had it for a long time and they have tried all the regular things. A good cure for dandruff is the tea tree oil shampoo, it's very, very good, also (evening) primrose oil, even in primrose oil capsules and an anti-oxidant tablet three times a day and you will cure 99 per cent of dandruff.[0]

■ Mix 25 drops of tea tree oil with 50 ml of slightly warmed jojoba or coconut oil and massage thoroughly into scalp. Wrap in warm towels and leave for an hour if possible. Wash out using a 3 per cent tea tree shampoo (about 5 drops of tea tree oil to 1 tsp of a mild shampoo) – apply the shampoo first before the water, otherwise the hair will remain oily. Repeat once a week.

■ Use a 2–3 per cent tea tree shampoo on a daily or regular basis (see instructions page 29).

- A quick method to use between washes, if required, is to rub a few drops of pure tea tree oil into the scalp using the fingertips.

See also **Hair Care**

Dermatitis/Eczema

Dermatitis and eczema are general terms used to describe a variety of inflamed or irritated skin conditions characterized by redness, flaky skin, rashes and itching, which in turn can lead to blisters, weepy sores and scabs.

The cause of the problem can vary – though many forms of dermatitis are associated with hereditary allergic tendencies, especially to certain foods (notably dairy or wheat products). Another form, known as contact dermatitis, is the result of the skin's hypersensitivity to an external irritant such as a type of detergent or cosmetic, or to dust, wool or some other substance. It is often very difficult to identify the cause, because the reaction may appear some time after the initial contact, or the skin may suddenly react adversely to a familiar substance. In all cases, however, mental stress or other emotional factors tend to aggravate or trigger an attack.

Tea tree has been found to be very effective for many types of dermatitis including militaria (prickly heat), nettle rash (*see* **Hives**), dust mites and rashes due to poison ivy or poison oak. In one dramatic case, an Australian man contracted such a severe cement dust allergy that the skin on his feet and calves became so tender and sore that the doctor had advised amputation of both legs below the knee! Then his wife saw a programme about tea tree oil on the television:

I purchased a bottle from my health food shop and we rubbed it all over the affected area. Within 2 weeks the condition had cleared up totally and now 11 months later there has been no recurrence whatsoever.[9]

NOTE

It may be necessary to experiment with different essential oils and types of treatment due to the individual nature of these types of skin problems. Always check carefully for sensitization or any type of allergic reaction before treating dermatitis using tea tree oil (see Safety Data, pages 31–2, for instructions on how to carry out a patch test).

- Apply pure tea tree oil to the affected area.
- For larger areas, make up a 1 per cent tea tree gel or non-oily cream (see instructions page 29) and apply to the affected area twice daily.
- Add 8–10 drops of tea tree oil to the bath water.
- Other measures: try to identify and remove possible causes of irritation; assess and improve the emotional environment if possible; the essential oils of chamomile, lavender, melissa, neroli and bergamot (bergapten-free) are also beneficial for skin complaints of this type – either used individually or in combination, employed in the bath or in creams/gels.

Dhobi Itch

Dhobi itch is a fungal infection caused by *Tinea cruris*. It usually affects men and is especially common during the summer or in hot climates. Inflamed pimples appear on the inside of the upper thigh and then merge to form a scaly, red and itchy patch with a clearly marked edge.

- Wash and dry the affected area thoroughly and apply neat tea tree twice a day.
- Avoid tight, synthetic clothing and allow the area to 'breathe' as much as possible.

See also **Tinea**

Disinfectant Uses

Tea tree has excellent antiseptic properties and as such it can be used very effectively as a disinfectant for first-aid purposes as well as for more general household chores. It is ideal for treating cuts, bites, burns, etc., for unlike many other disinfectant lotions it does not sting exposed skin. A dilute water solution can be used for swabbing down washable surfaces, and a few drops added to the laundry water will disinfect nappies (diapers), clothes, towels, etc. The vaporized oil can also be used very effectively to disinfect rooms at home or in the workplace, especially during or following infectious illness. Tea tree oil is already being used commercially to control bacteria and fungi via air-conditioning systems. After using a tea tree product in this manner, one firm claimed 'a marked reduction in absenteeism due to sickness such as colds and flu', while another noted that tea tree 'eliminated mould growth and its unsightly wall stains, unacceptable musty smell and damage to wallpaper, paintwork and furnishings'.[10]

It was tested as a germicide in Australia in 1980 in a solution of only 4 parts essential oil to 1,000 parts water with great success. According to one Australian doctor it will only be a matter of time before tea tree oil becomes 'ubiquitous' throughout the household:

> ... you put a bit of tea tree disinfectant in the washing water when you are washing your clothes and things like that ... It is going to be the antiseptic of the future.[11]

Researchers at the University of Sydney have also shown that tea tree oil when added to the wash at normal temperatures will kill dust mites – the cause of numerous allergic reactions, being especially harmful to asthma sufferers.

> Their experiments showed that a 0.8 per cent solution (80 ml per 10 litres of water) of tea tree oil in the wash killed all the mites after 30 minutes and almost 80 per cent after 10 minutes.[12]

> ■ Disinfecting clothes, nappies (diapers), etc.: for hand washing, add up to 50 drops of tea tree oil to half a litre of warm water; otherwise add up to 50 drops to a liquid detergent before putting into the washing machine.

- For washing floors, surfaces, etc.: add up to 50 drops to a bucket or bowl of water and stir well before mopping or wiping surfaces.
- For cleaning cuts, wounds, etc.: add a few drops of neat tea tree to a small bowl of cooled boiled water and swab the damaged area using a cotton wool or gauze pad.
- Disinfecting sickrooms, bathrooms, workplaces, etc.: diffuse tea tree into the air – for various methods see page 30.
- There are many other oils which also have excellent disinfectant properties, including lavender, lemon, eucalyptus, thyme and bergamot.

Eczema

– see **Dermatitis/Eczema**

Fever

A raised temperature is a vital and healthy response to infection because it speeds up the body's metabolic rate and strengthens its natural defense systems.

In many instances a fever should be allowed to take its course – a process which often culminates in a period of profuse sweating which eventually subsides together with a lowering of the fever.

Tea tree oil is a very useful aid for feverish conditions, involving infection due to its powerful anti-viral, bactericidal and immuno-stimulant qualities. Tea tree oil can also help to induce perspiration when the body needs to 'sweat it out', due to its diaphoretic properties (although it does not cause sweating when the body is in a normal state).

NOTE

If the fever remains high, or rises to a dangerous level, seek professional medical advice immediately.

- Use tea tree in vaporizers throughout the duration of the illness, but especially at the onset. In addition, add a few drops to a handkerchief for inhalation throughout the day, and to the pillow for night use.
- To help control a high temperature, immerse the whole body in a tepid bath containing 3–10 drops (depending on the person's age) of tea tree oil.
- If the person is too weak to get into a bath, sponge his or her body down using a flannel (wash-cloth) soaked in tepid water to which a few drops of tea tree oil have been added.
- Other measures: drink plenty of pure water or liquids to detoxify the system and prevent dehydration. Other essential oils of benefit include peppermint, eucalyptus, bergamot and lavender.

See also **Bronchitis, Chickenpox, Flu, Measles, Sinusitis**

Flu

Influenza is the most common single cause of fever, although the term is often used to include various unidentified viral infections characterized by a raised temperature, aching limbs, fatigue, a sore throat and other respiratory symptoms such as catarrh or a dry cough.

Self-help using essential oils can do much to prevent an attack of flu, or at least to reduce the severity of the illness, the most effective being tea tree.

- Use tea tree in vaporizers throughout the duration of the illness, but especially at the onset of flu – this may prevent it from developing at all. In addition, add a few drops to a handkerchief for inhalation throughout the day, and to the pillow for night use.
- At the very first sign of infection take a hot bath adding 8–10 drops of tea tree to the water – then go straight to bed. Repeat each evening, or every other night – this is often enough to avert a full-blown attack.
- For a sore throat, add 5–10 drops of tea tree to a glass of warm water, mix well and gargle. Repeat 2 or 3 times a day at least.
- For a cough, make up a concentrated chest rub by mixing 5 drops of tea tree with 5 drops of marjoram (or benzoin) in 1 dessertspoon of carrier oil and apply to the chest and upper back. Repeat at least twice a day.
- To relieve congestion, add 5–6 drops of tea tree oil to a bowl of steaming water, cover your head with towel and breathe deeply for

5–10 minutes with your eyes closed ... very hot steam is in itself a
hostile environment for viruses. Repeat at least twice a day.
- Other measures: take a course of garlic capsules. Lavender, marjoram or chamomile oil can also be used in baths to soothe aching limbs and encourage restful sleep.

See also **Colds, Coughs, Fever, Sinusitis, Sore Throat**

Genital Herpes

Genital herpes is an infection transmitted by sexual contact, caused by the virus *herpes simplex II.* The first attack is generally the worst; the skin of the genital region becomes red and itchy and then erupts into small, very painful blisters which can last for several weeks. This tends to be followed by recurrent attacks which take a milder form and which are often precipitated by stress, sexual activity or another infection; these subsequent attacks usually last only a few days. Nevertheless, genital herpes remains a very distressing condition that does not respond to standard antibiotic treatment (like cold sores, which are also caused by herpes simplex and also do not respond to antibiotics). Due to its powerful anti-viral action, however, tea tree oil has been found to be of great value in treating this stubborn problem.[13]

- At the very first sign of infection make a concentrated solution by mixing 30 drops of tea tree oil with about 1 litre of warm water – shake or stir well before use. Use this solution to douche or wash the genital area frequently to soothe irritation and prevent the infection from developing.

- *Note:* Although it is normal to experience a temporary, warm sensation, discontinue this method if irritation occurs.
- Use neat tea tree oil to dab any blisters as soon as they begin to develop – check for sensitivity first! Repeat frequently over a period of several days, or until the condition has cleared.
- Add 8–10 drops to the bath water as a general disinfectant measure.
- Other measures: any sexual partners should also undergo treatment to avoid re-infection; abstain from sexual contact for at least a week during the treatment; take vitamin C tablets; lavender and bergamot (bergapten-free) oil are also beneficial for treating genital herpes when applied in the same manner as tea tree.

See also **Cold Sores, Zona (Shingles)**

Gingivitis

– see **Mouth and Gum Infections**

Gout

– see **Arthritis**

Hair Care

Tea tree oil makes an excellent conditioning treatment for the hair due to its fresh scent, gentle action and powerful antiseptic properties. It helps to regulate the activity of the sebaceous glands, cleanses the scalp of bacterial and fungal infection and helps disperse dead skin cells. By making the hair more healthy and manageable, tea tree oil benefits all hair types including dry hair, greasy hair and itchy scalp conditions.

- Choose a mild or pH neutral shampoo which does not strip the hair of its protective acid mantle, then add between 1 and 2 per cent of tea tree oil (about 20–50 drops per 100 ml of mild shampoo – or 2–3 drops of tea tree oil to 1 tsp of shampoo). Shampoo daily or according to your usual routine – this treatment is good for all hair types. (A more concentrated solution is required for treating dandruff).

- Tea tree oil can also be added to a conditioning lotion in the same manner (2 per cent), or a few drops can be put in the final rinse water.

- Hair conditioner: mix 25 drops of tea tree oil with 50 ml of slightly warmed jojoba or coconut oil, massage thoroughly into scalp. Wrap hair in a warm towel and leave for an hour if possible. Wash out, using tea tree shampoo – apply the shampoo first before the water, otherwise the hair will remain oily. Repeat once a week. (Alternatively, a few drops of tea tree oil can be added to natural conditioning lotion or wax).

- A good final rinse for all hair types is to add 5 drops of tea tree and 1 tbsp of cider vinegar to the final rinse water. This will help to remove detergent residue and restore the acid equilibrium of the scalp.
- Various other essential oils are also beneficial for the hair including chamomile, lavender and rosemary.

See also **Cradle Cap, Dandruff, Lice, Ringworm**

Halitosis (Bad Breath)

– see **Mouth and Gum Infections**

Hives (Nettle Rash/Urticaria)

Hives are an allergic eruption of the skin characterized by a burning, itchy sensation and the appearance of red bumps, blotches or small boils – similar to a nettle sting. In severe cases they may appear as large red weals. This type of allergic reaction can be triggered by a number of different factors, such as the consumption of a certain food or in response to an external irritant such as dust – stress is often another aggravating factor.

For methods of treatment see **Dermatitis**

Immune System (to Strengthen)

The immune response is orchestrated by three distinct groups of cells — the phagocytes, the 'T' cells and 'B' cells. These all originate from white blood cells in the bone marrow and serve to protect the body from infection. If this defensive barrier is damaged for some reason, the body becomes vulnerable to invasion from all sorts of pathogenic organisms. The immune system is supported by and closely related to other body functions, especially the lymphatic and nervous systems. Recent research tends to suggest that emotional and psychological factors play a vital role in the efficiency of the immune response.[14] This may help to account for the fact that viral infections and suppressed immune systems are becoming an increasing problem today — while diseases such as AIDS, Chronic Fatigue Syndrome (ME) and other viral infections are presenting symptoms not previously encountered.

Many essential oils, particularly tea tree oil, are very beneficial used in this context since they can assist the body in resisting and fighting infection:

1. by directly opposing the threatening micro-organisms.

2. by stimulating and increasing the activity of the organs and cells involved.

3. by building up resistance and promoting the immune system as a whole.

As a preventative measure, tea tree is already being used to increase the immune response of patients before surgery and to build up the strength of those suffering from long-term debilitating illnesses such as glandular fever, hepatitis and Chronic Fatigue Syndrome. The value of tea tree in slowing down the development and furthering the treatment of AIDS is also undergoing investigation with some success.[15]

- To help build up resistance levels, take a bath at least twice a week using 8–10 drops of tea tree oil in the water.
- To strengthen the immune system, have a massage once a week using a 2.5 per cent tea tree oil blend (see instructions pages 28–9). If this is not possible, make up a 5 per cent concentrated massage oil blend and rub this firmly into the palms of the hands and soles of the feet once a day.
- Use tea tree and other essential oils as room fragrances on an everyday basis.
- Other measures: a course of garlic capsules, vitamin E and vitamin C are also indicated.

Impetigo

This highly infectious skin disease which mainly affects children is usually caused by an invasion of the *streptococcus* or *staphylococcus* bacteria. Inflamed patches or spots appear, usually on the face, scalp and neck, but sometimes on the hands and knees – which blister and then crust over.

The bactericidal action of tea tree makes it very effective in treating this contagious skin condition. Strict hygiene is also essential to prevent the condition from spreading to other parts of the body – or to other people. An Australian herbal practitioner who uses tea tree in his practice writes:

> Tea tree works really well with ... impetigo, the herpes simplex blisters and most types of ulcerous tissue ... it replaces anti-biotic infection, irritation and discomfort.[16]

- Apply pure tea tree oil to the affected area, using the tip of the finger or a cotton bud (swab). Repeat twice a day.
- Add 10 drops (no more than 5 for children) to the bath water as a disinfectant measure.
- Lavender oil may also be used to treat impetigo.

Insect Bites/Stings

For a long time tea tree oil has been used in Australia for the treatment of a variety of insect bites and stings. It has been found to bring fast relief from the bites of mosquitoes, sandflies, fleas and horseflies, and from wasp and bee stings, as well as some types of spider and jellyfish! Dabbed directly onto the bite, tea tree not only soothes itching and relieves pain, it also prevents any infection from developing due to scratching – especially among children.

One woman was concerned for her son who on returning from summer camp was covered with mosquito bites:

He was scratching them, making matters worse. I applied tea tree oil and in just 20 minutes the itching stopped and the next morning all was well.[17]

Another woman reported how after returning from a trip to Dubai she suffered from several mosquito bites on her legs which were causing inflammation and suppuration:

I bathed in this [tea tree oil], 10 drops to a bath, and also separately bathed the wounds ... I had an immediate reaction and relief and the swelling was reduced.[18]

Because tea tree is an effective antiseptic yet gentle on the skin, it can be used over and over again with little fear of causing irritation. Tea tree oil also makes an excellent insect repellant – a discovery made by the early tea tree cutters.

- To treat bites and stings apply neat tea tree oil to the affected area – repeat every 4 hours or as required.
- 5–10 drops added to the bath water is also beneficial.
- As a preventative measure, tea tree oil can be applied neat to exposed skin; to clothing such as socks, scarves, etc.; or diluted in a light vegetable oil base for application to larger areas.
- To keep insects out of the house, apply tea tree to hanging ribbons or use a vaporizer.

- Other measures: there are several oils which have insect-repellant properties, the most useful being lavender, citronella, lemongrass, eucalyptus or atlas cedarwood – or a combination of these.

Leucorrhoea/Pruritis

Leucorrhoea is an inflammation of the vagina caused by a proliferation of unwanted bacteria or fungi, which can have a variety of causes. Symptoms often include a thick white or yellow discharge and severe itching of the vaginal area.

Pruritis or itching is an irritating condition which generally accompanies any type of mild vaginal infection, such as trichomonal vaginitis or cervicitis.

Tea tree has been found to be very effective for the treatment of all these conditions:

> It will help relieve the itch from the genital wart virus, from candida, and from non-specific bacterial or fungal infection. It will relieve the symptoms as well as overcoming the infections so ... treating the cause of the problem.[19]

- As a sitz bath, add 8–10 drops of tea tree oil to a bowl or shallow bath of warm water and soak for 5 10 minutes.
- Bathe daily, adding 8–10 drops of tea tree to the bath water as a general antiseptic measure.

- Make up a 1 per cent tea tree ointment – using a hypo-allergenic bland cream base (see instructions pages 29–30). Apply to the affected area as required.
- In addition, avoid tight clothing, nylon underwear and harsh bubble baths; take garlic capsules and keep tea, coffee, alcohol and spices to a minimum; other oils of benefit include lavender, bergamot and sandalwood.

See also **Cystitis, Thrush**

Lice (Pediculosis)

Lice are small blood-sucking insects which cause the scalp to become itchy and uncomfortable; they are a common and recurrent problem among schoolchildren. Most establishments suffer from outbreaks from time to time since lice can pass very quickly from one head of hair to the next irrespective of hair type. The lice also lay tiny greyish-white eggs (nits) which attach themselves firmly to the hair, usually near to the scalp.

Both lice and eggs are quite hard to see and can be difficult to remove. Tea tree oil kills lice, but not their eggs, so it must be used regularly until all the eggs have either hatched or been removed. Although the tea tree remedy requires more persistence than commercial chemical treatments, it actually improves the quality of the hair rather than damaging it.

- At the start of an outbreak use a 2–3 per cent tea tree oil shampoo on a daily basis to prevent contamination (see instructions page 29).
- Another tip for lice prevention is eating a garlic pearl once a day.
- If lice or eggs are found on the hair, make up an alcohol-based scalp rub by adding 5 ml of tea tree to 25 ml of vodka mixed with 75 ml water – leave on for at least an hour (overnight if possible), then wash out. Finally, comb the hair carefully with a fine-toothed comb. Use this preparation at the start of an infestation and repeat every 3 days until the condition has cleared up. Two or three applications will usually do the trick! (Replace the alcohol/water mix with a vegetable oil if the skin becomes irritated).
- Between treatments, wash the hair daily (if possible) with a 2–3 per cent tea tree shampoo – leave on for 10 minutes before washing out. In addition add a little tea tree oil to the conditioner or final rinse water.
- To prevent reinfection, wash all combs and brushes in water to which a few drops of tea tree oil have been added.
- Other measures: lavender oil is also an effective remedy for lice.

Measles

Measles is a viral infection characterized by a sore throat, a barking cough, sensitivity to light and a blotchy rash usually starting on the face and neck and spreading to the trunk and limbs. A doctor should always be consulted since measles, especially in adults, can lead to complications – though the following measures can do much to ensure that the attack is mild and of short duration.

- If the fever is very high it can be reduced by applying cold compresses, sponging the body down at regular intervals or, if possible, by immersing the whole body in a luke warm bath to which a few drops of tea tree oil have been added.
- Use tea tree in vaporizers in and around the sick room for the course of the illness, to prevent the development and spread of infection.
- Regular steam inhalations will help to soothe coughing – add 5 drops of tea tree to a bowl of steaming hot water and inhale for 5–10 minutes, keeping the eyes closed.
- For the treatment of a sore throat add 5–10 drops of tea tree oil to a glass of warm water, mix well, and gargle.

See also **Fever, Sore Throat**

Moniliasis

– *see* **Candida**

Mouth and Gum Infections

There are several types of mouth and gum infections, having different causes. The most common are:

a Mouth ulcers – tiny blisters which then burst to form ulcers (2–10 mm in diameter) on the tongue, under the tongue or on the inside of the cheeks.

b Candidiasis (or thrush) of the mouth, which is common among young children but also sometimes in adults especially after a course of antibiotics. It is caused by the fungal infection *Candida albicans*, the same organism that causes vaginal thrush. Oral thrush appears as small white flecks on the inside of the cheeks or roof of the mouth – the breath is also often offensive.

c Gingivitis – a red spongy swelling of the gums, making them bleed easily, especially when cleaning the teeth. The condition is aggravated by poor dental care and hygiene. Studies have shown that washing the mouth out twice a day with a tea tree solution will inhibit the growth of bacteria, reduce gum bleeding and help control plaque.[20] (See page 9).

■ For candidiasis (thrush) or mouth ulcers, dilute tea tree to 50 per cent in water, mix well and apply to the spots or ulcers with a cotton bud (swab) – repeat twice daily for 3 days. To reduce the strong taste for young children, dilute 1 drop of tea tree in some of the child's saliva before application.

■ For the treatment of gingivitis and bad breath (halitosis) or other mouth and gum infections, add 5–10 drops of tea tree oil to a glass of warm water, mix well, rinse the mouth and/or gargle on a daily or twice daily basis. Repeat each morning and evening after brushing the teeth.

■ Alternatively, make up a 5 per cent tea tree and water solution spray, and use as required.

Muscular Aches and Pains

Muscular aches and pains are a common affliction caused either by physical over-exertion or by psychological stress and strain. Many people, for example, carry tension in their necks and shoulders which over a period of time causes the muscles to become tight and painful.

■ Soaking in a hot bath is an easy and effective way of relaxing the muscles and bringing instant pain relief ... 8–10 drops of tea tree oil added to the water will increase the benefits further due to its analgesic (pain-killing) and penetrative qualities.

■ Muscular aches and pains respond well to local massage – add about 9 drops of tea tree to 1 tbsp of carrier oil and rub into the affected area.

■ To relieve muscular spasm or if a particular area is very tight, massage with neat tea tree oil or apply a hot compress to which a few drops of tea tree oil have been added.

■ A few drops of tea tree rubbed into the muscles before and immediately after strenuous sport can help prevent muscular aches and pains from developing.

- Other oils of benefit include lavender, marjoram, rosemary, black pepper and chamomile.

Nails (Infected)

– *see* **Paronychia**

Nappy (Diaper) Rash

A common complaint among babies, nappy rash is often a form of dermatitis or eczema caused by the skin's reaction to the acid in urine. However, some forms of nappy rash are due to a candida (thrush) infection contracted while passing through the birth canal.

- Nappy rash – soothe by adding 1 drop of tea tree to 1 tsp of baby cream and applying at each nappy change.
- Prevent re-infection by using 3 drops (1 drop for babies under 18 months) of tea tree diluted in 1 tsp vegetable oil regularly in baths, and by adding a few drops of tea tree to water used for washing nappies, towels and baby clothes.
- Other essential oils of benefit include chamomile and lavender.

See also **Candida**

Paronychia

Paronychia is a fungal infection affecting the fingernails and toenails. The cuticle becomes red and painful with a slight discharge, and the skin beneath the nail becomes discoloured; eventually the nail itself becomes furrowed and distorted. It is often caused by contact with harsh detergents or by applying false nails on a regular basis.

Although the infection penetrates deep under the nail, tea tree is very effective in treating this stubborn affliction because of its penetrating fungicidal properties.[21]

> ■ Soak the infected nails in pure tea tree oil for 2 or 3 minutes, massaging the solution into the nailbed. Repeat 3 times a day until the infection clears.

Pets/Animal Care

Essential oils are increasingly employed for the treatment of common ailments in veterinary practice and for the care of domestic pets – particularly dogs, cats and horses.

NOTE

Care should be taken in using neat tea tree on small animals, due to its high concentration.

- Fleas – use tea tree shampoo (see instructions page 29) on a daily basis – leave for 3–5 minutes before washing out. Afterwards or between washes wipe the coat with a moist sponge sprinkled with 10–20 drops of pure oil. This also improves the condition of the coat.

- Lice – sprinkle the coat with 10–20 drops of tea tree oil and brush thoroughly. Repeat daily.

- Ticks – apply pure tea tree oil directly onto the tick, then remove. Continue to apply the oil 2–3 times a day to any tick bites until they have healed.

- Rashes – apply pure tea tree oil or, if needed to treat a larger area, use tea tree diluted to 2.5 per cent with a light carrier oil or cream (see instructions pages 29–30).

- Cuts/itches/scabs/insect bites/bumps – apply pure tea tree oil. Repeat 2–3 times a day until healed.

- Fungal disease affecting fish – add 1 or 2 drops (depending on the size of the tank or pond) of tea tree to the water once every day for a week.

- Other measures: lavender oil may be used in a similar fashion.

Pruritis (Itching)

– *see* **Leucorrhoea/Pruritis**

Psoriasis

Psoriasis is a non-contagious skin disease which varies enormously in its severity and frequency of occurrence. Common symptoms include chronic scaling, plaques, ringed lesions, smooth red areas and acute pustules.

Psoriasis is believed to be caused by a dysfunction of skin enzymes together with an increased turnover of epidermal cells and a dilation of dermal capillaries. The condition can be precipitated by mental stress and is often associated with a deep-seated emotional disturbance of some kind. Symptomatic treatment is therefore best carried out alongside a psychological approach or exploration of possible causes and contributing factors. Food allergies, vitamin deficiency and environmental influences can also contribute to this distressing condition.

Due to the factors mentioned above, psoriasis is a difficult condition to treat and may involve a variety of different approaches. On a symptomatic level, however, tea tree oil, cajuput and myrrh have been used with considerable success in alleviating the problem.

- Make up a thick lotion by blending 50 ml avocado oil and 50 ml borage seed (or Evening Primrose Oil) with a little wheatgerm oil, then add 30 drops of tea tree and 10 drops each of cajuput and myrrh essential oils. Apply at least twice daily to the affected area.
- Other measures: using Dead Sea salt in baths and exposing the skin to sunlight are also beneficial in some cases.

Rheumatism

The term 'rheumatism' is used medically to describe a whole range of disorders which involve pain in the muscles or joints, including the various forms of arthritis and gout. Generally speaking, however, rheumatism refers specifically to muscular pain, whereas arthritis and gout are associated with pain located within the joints themselves.

Tea tree can help to ease rheumatic pain due to its analgesic qualities – it also increases local blood circulation and enhances mobility. Since rheumatism, like arthritis, is aggravaged by an accumulation of toxins in the system, the diet and lifestyle should also be assessed.

- Massage is itself very helpful for rheumatic pains because it stimulates the circulation and helps remove toxins. Make up a concentrated massage oil by mixing 30 drops of tea tree oil with 50 ml of a vegetable carrier oil. Apply twice daily.
- Add 8–10 drops of tea tree oil to the bath water for pain relief.
- For this complaint, tea tree is best used in combination with other oils including chamomile, lavender, marjoram and rosemary.

See also **Arthritis, Muscular Aches and Pains**

Ringworm

A number of different fungal organisms may be responsible for ringworm, but in its most common form it affects the scalp (*Tinea capitis*) causing scaly skin and itching – temporary bald patches may also appear.

Tea tree oil is very effective at treating the Tinea fungus in all its various forms, and usually only takes a few days to take effect:

- Make up a 5 per cent tea tree cream, gel or oil (see pages 29–30) and apply 3–4 times a day to the affected skin. Alternatively, neat tea tree can be applied directly to small areas in the same way.
- For ringworm of the scalp, apply the tea tree treatment in the same manner, then wash the hair daily with a tea tree shampoo (see instructions page 29).
- To help restore hair growth after the infection has disappeared, replace the tea tree oil with rosemary essential oil in a 5 per cent cream and massage this into the bald patch. Additionally use a rosemary shampoo, and mix a few drops of rosemary oil into the final rinse water.
- Add 8–10 drops to the bath water as an additional treatment.
- Combs, brushes, clothes, bedding, etc. should be disinfected by adding a few drops of tea tree oil to the washing water.
- Other oils of benefit which may be used in combination with tea tree include lavender and myrrh.

See also **Disinfectant Uses, Tinea**

Scabies

Scabies is a highly contagious skin disease caused by the itch mite *sarcoptes scabiei*. Scabies is common in sheepfarming areas, where it is commonly transmitted from the wool of the sheep to the farm workers. It can also be picked up in changing rooms, and even from handling coins – it does not require close contact to pass from one person to another. The female mites lay their eggs under the skin, and as the newly hatched mites burrow their way out this causes severe irritation and itching – especially at night. Small red pimples may appear and scratching can lead to sores which can then become infected. Common areas to be affected are the groin, penis, nipples and the skin between the fingers.

- Wash the skin gently, then treat the affected area with a 5 per cent tea tree non-oily cream or gel (see instructions pages 29–30) – repeat 2 or 3 times a day.
- As a matter of routine, add 8–10 drops of tea tree to the bath water as a disinfectant measure.
- During treatment scrupulous attention to hygiene is essential. To prevent re-infection, change and wash pillowcases, towels, bedding, clothes (especially woollens), etc. using a few drops of tea tree oil in the washing water – sponge the mattress down using a 10 per cent solution in alcohol.
- Other oils of benefit: lavender, peppermint.

Shingles

– *see* Zona

Sinusitis

Sinusitis is an infection of the mucous membranes lining the body cavities behind, above and on either side of the nose. It usually follows a cold, hayfever or prolonged exposure to cold, damp air. An acute attack is often accompanied by congested headaches and catarrh, sometimes with fever. Chronic or long-term sinusitis indicates a mild infection which causes the nose to be continually blocked and a dull pain or feeling of tension to manifest in the area between the eyes. People who suffer from constant or repeated attacks of sinusitis often suffer from allergies – especially to gluten and cow's milk.

NOTE

Sinusitis can lead to secondary infections, notably ear infections and very occasionally meningitis – if in doubt seek professional advice immediately.

■ Steam inhalations relieve congestion and fight infection – use 5 drops of tea tree oil in a bowl of steaming water, cover your head with a towel, and inhale deeply for 5–10 minutes with your eyes closed. Repeat several times a day.

■ Use 8–10 drops in the bath water – this acts as a kind of steam inhalation.

- Use tea tree oil in a vaporizer in the bedroom at night – or put a few drops on the pillow. Tea tree can also be applied to a handkerchief for use throughout the day.
- A course of garlic capsules is also indicated.
- Certain foods, especially dairy produce (made from cow's milk) and wheat products aggravate the problem and should be eliminated from the diet as much as possible during treatment.
- Other essential oils of benefit for congestion include eucalyptus, niaouli and peppermint (used in vaporizers or steam inhalation).

See also **Colds, Fever**

Skin Care

Tea tree is a valuable skin care agent because although it has excellent antiseptic properties it is very mild on the skin. As such it can be used for a wide range of specific skin conditions as well as for more general disinfectant purposes. In a theoretical comparison between tea tree and other antiseptics used for skin care, tea tree oil came closest to having all the properties of 'an ideal skin disinfectant'. This is because it:

1 has a rapid bactericidal action against a wide range of organisms with good persistence and with the added attribute of a high degree of absorption into the derma

2 possesses marked cleaning properties noted repeatedly in clinical literature

3 does not irritate the skin, is not poisonous, does not harm tissue cells, and has no significant side-effects

4 is not easily contaminated

5 is cosmetically very suitable, being colourless and of a pleasant, clean odour

6 is nearly neutral in pH

7 is notably effective in the presence of organic detritus (dirt, blood and pus)

8 is notably effective on fungi, and is used on viral complaints with success.[22]

In addition, tea tree is not only beneficial for blemished or oily complexions but also for those people whose skin is prone to dehydration. In other words, it is suitable for all skin types.

- As a cleaner/toner for everyday skin care, but especially for those with problem (blemished/oily) skin, blend 15 drops each of tea tree and lavender essential oils with 25 ml of witchhazel and 75 ml distilled water (or another flower water) and apply morning and night before moisturizing the skin.

- For moisturizing the skin, blend 3 drops of tea tree with 1 tsp wheatgerm oil (or a moisturizing cream); apply twice daily.

See also Acne, Cracked Skin, Dermatitis/Eczema, Hives, Psoriasis

Sore Throat

A sore throat often accompanies other respiratory infections such as flu, bronchitis, tonsilitis and the common cold. It is often the first sign of illness, and if treated immediately can prevent further infection from developing – or at least shorten the duration of the disease ...

> came down with sore throats; we gargled with few drops [of tea tree] in water and within a few days the sore throat was gone.[23]

■ Add 5–10 drops of tea tree oil to a glass of warm water, mix well and gargle at least 2 or 3 times a day. Continue until the condition has cleared up.

■ Other oils of benefit: sage, thyme.

Splinters, Infected

After removing a splinter, always apply a drop of tea tree oil to prevent infection. Splinters can be dangerous if they do become infected – often because a small portion of the splinter remains embedded in the skin.

■ If the splinter is infected, sore and with pus: clean the area gently, apply pure tea tree oil, then cover with a clay poultice or plaster (adhesive bandage) and leave for 2 hours to help draw it out.

Remove the splinter with a pair of tweezers – repeat the procedure if this does not work – then apply a few drops of tea tree and cover with a plaster (adhesive bandage).

■ Other oils of benefit: lavender, chamomile (for inflammation).

Spots

– see **Acne**

Sunburn

Tea tree oil is a very useful oil to have in hot climates – not least because it is excellent for sunburn. If applied immediately, tea tree lotion can provide instant relief from heat rash or red and sore skin – it can also prevent blistering.

■ For large areas, make up a lotion using 12 drops of tea tree oil in 1 tbsp of distilled water (or a water-based gel to which 5–10 per cent tea tree oil has been added) and dab the area gently.

■ For severe patches of sunburn apply tea tree oil neat.

■ Other measures: soaking in a lukewarm bath containing 6–8 drops of tea tree or chamomile roman is very soothing; lavender is also a very effective sunburn remedy when used in the same manner as tea tree.

See also **Burns**

Sweaty Feet

Tea tree is an excellent disinfectant and deodorant – with a fresh, pleasing scent.

- Add 5–10 drops of tea tree to a bowl of warm water and soak the feet nightly for 5 minutes.
- As a quick measure, a few drops of tea tree oil can be rubbed into the soles of the feet in the morning.

Throat

– see **Sore Throat**

Thrush

Thrush is caused by a yeast-like fungus called *Candida albicans* (formerly known as *Monilia albicans*). This organism is present in the body naturally, only causing problems when it proliferates above a certain level. Some people are more prone to such an infection than others, and this can be connected to food allergies, low immunity levels, stress and, quite commonly, as a result of antibiotic treatment. This is because antibiotics, as well as attacking germs, also kill some of the intestinal flora which generally keep the candida organisms under control.

In women the most common site of infection is in the vagina, where the symptoms of this irritating condition include severe itching, redness and often a milky-white discharge. Tea tree is very effective for treating this distressing condition.[24]

Although it is normal to experience a temporary, warm sensation when tea tree is used in the vaginal area, discontinue treatment if a burning irritation develops.

- A simple way of treating vaginal thrush is to soak a tampon in a 1 per cent solution of tea tree oil in purified or distilled water (20 drops to 100 ml water). Insert into the vagina and replace every 24 hours. (This is the routine method employed at the Annandale Women's Centre, Sydney, Australia).

- Alternatively, vaginal pessaries can be made using a 2 per cent dilution of tea tree oil in a cocoa butter base – warm the cocoa butter slightly, add the tea tree, form into pellets then leave to harden. These can be inserted into the vagina on a daily basis.

- For a vaginal douche or enema add 10 drops of oil to half a litre (500 ml) of purified or distilled water – this helps to reduce infection, irritation and discomfort, and may be used between those times when you need the above methods of treatment.

- As a sitz bath, add 8–10 drops of tea tree oil to a bowl or shallow bath of warm water and soak for 5–10 minutes.

- Bathe daily adding 8–10 drops of tea tree to the bath water as a general precautionary measure.

- To avoid re-infection, any sexual partners should undergo treatment simultaneously. Balanitis (a candida infection of the penis) may be treated by washing the area carefully with a 1 per cent solution of tea tree in distilled water (20 drops to 100 ml water) applied 4 times a day.

■ In addition, during treatment it is advisable to eat plenty of live yogurt, take acidophilus capsules, avoid alcohol and keep sugary and starchy foods to a minimum. For those who recurrently suffer bouts of thrush, the diet may need to be adjusted on a more permanent basis.

See also **Candida**

Ticks and Leeches

Tea tree oil can be used to repel ticks and leeches – the early tea tree cutters applied tea tree to their socks to ward off leeches which were common in the swampy Australian coastal regions! If they do manage to attach themselves to the skin, these blood-sucking parasites are notoriously difficult to remove – tea tree is also a great aid in this respect.

■ Apply neat tea tree oil to the live tick or leech as well as the surrounding skin and leave on for at least 20 minutes. Carefully remove by hand those ticks or leeches which have not already fallen off.

■ Continue to apply the neat oil to the tick/leech bites 3 times a day for a week to soothe any irritation and prevent possible infection.

Tinea

Tinea is caused by a microscopic fungal mould which manifests in several forms, though all are characterized by red, flaky skin and itching. Athlete's foot is caused by *Tinea pedis*; ringworm generally by *Tinea capitis*; (nicknamed 'dhobi itch') affects the groin (especially in hot climates); and *Tinea barbae*, sometimes known as 'barber's rash', affects the face and neck.

For treatment see **Athlete's Foot, Barber's Rash, Dhobi Itch, Ringworm**

Tonsilitis

– *see* **Sore Throat**

Ulcers (Varicose and Tropical)

Varicose ulcers can form on the lower legs when the veins are not functioning properly, often as a result of varicose veins. Elderly people are particularly prone to this condition, especially if they suffer from poor circulation – some merely have to scratch the skin on their lower legs to develop a sore which can be very slow to heal.

Tropical ulcers (also known as 'naga sores') usually occur in hot, humid climates. Again a large painless sore develops, often on the feet or legs, due to a bacterial infection, poor nutrition or environmental factors.

Tea tree has been found to be very effective at preventing and treating ulcers of the lower limbs. Moisturizing the skin of this area with tea tree oil cream every day is very good as it keeps the skin moist, and it also prevents the infection of little abrasions:

Many cases of extreme ulcerations of the legs, with considerable suppurations, which have not responded to treatment by any other means, have been quickly cured by treatment with Ti-trol [tea tree oil].[25]

- As a preventative measure, apply a 5 per cent tea tree cream/oil (see instructions pages 29–30) to the lower legs on a daily basis.
- To treat an ulcer, bathe the sore gently with a warm diluted solution of tea tree oil (by adding a few drops to a bowl of distilled/boiled water). Then apply a 10 per cent tea tree cream (see instructions pages 29–30), or cover with a pad which has been saturated in a solution of 3 parts olive oil to 1 part tea tree oil.
- Lavender oil is also a very effective treatment for ulcers when used in the same manner.

For mouth ulcers see **Mouth and Gum Infections**

Urethritis

– see **Cystitis/Urethritis**

Vaginal Infections

– see **Leucorrhoea/Pruritis, Thrush**

Warts/Veruccae

Warts are small (often hard) benign growths commonly occurring on the hands, fingers, face, elbows or knees. They are caused by a virus and are slightly contagious. They usually disappear of their own accord after some time, but because they are unsightly most people resort to a 'wart cure'. There are a great number of highly dubious folk remedies for warts, but the modern method is to burn them out or to apply a highly abrasive paste.

Plantar warts (*Verruca plantaris*) are also caused by a virus, and usually occur on the soles of the feet, often at the base of the toes. Small black dots are visible at the centre of the virus and, because of pressure on the feet, these warts can become painful.

Both types of wart are notoriously difficult to get rid of on a long-term basis, and the problem with the 'modern' types of cures is that they destroy all the surrounding healthy tissue as well as the wart and decrease the body's natural immunity, thereby increasing the potential for re-infection.

- Warts will often disappear if they are dabbed with neat tea tree oil 3 times a day. (It may take as long as a month or so to be effective, so a little perseverance is required!)

- Plantar warts or veruccae should be coated daily with a 50 per cent mixture of tea tree oil and myrrh resin, then covered with a plaster (adhesive bandage). After a few days, when the skin has gone yellowish and soggy, the black dots of the virus should be dug out with a needle or nail scissors – and the treatment continued (usually for about 6 weeks depending on the severity of the condition) until the skin has healed over.

Wounds

– *see* Cuts/Wounds

Zona (Shingles)

Zona is caused by the same virus as chickenpox – *herpes zoster*. The virus affects the sensory nerves, and causes clusters of blisters to appear, often in the form of a band around the torso. The condition can be accompanied by severe pain, usually before the rash appears, and there may be fever.

For treatment see Chickenpox

Further Information

PART THREE

Other Essential Oils
from the Tea Tree Group

TEA TREE OIL

Many of the 'tea tree' group of plants, apart from *Melaleuca alternifolia* produce essential oils which have shown some degree of healing properties. Hundreds have been analysed but only a few have attained commercial status. Notable among these are:

WHITE TEA TREE or Cajuput Tree (*Melaleuca cajuputi, M. minor*)

A graceful tree up to 14 m (45 ft) high in Southeast Asia, especially the Malay Peninsula as well as in Australia. In the East the essential oil is used as a popular household medicine and insecticide. Similar to niaouli oil, it contains principally cineole (50–65 per cent) – a possible skin irritant.

BROAD-LEAVED PAPERBARK TREE or Bellbowrie (*Melaleuca viridiflora, M. quinquenervia*)

A very tall vigorous tree up to 18 m (60 ft) high, found in Australia, Tasmania and the French Pacific Islands. The oil known as 'niaouli' or 'gomenol' is used locally as a disinfectant and as a medicine especially for its antiseptic properties.

Similar to cajuput oil, it contains principally cineole (50–65 per cent) – a possible skin irritant. Frequently subject to adulteration.

NARROW-LEAVED PAPERBARK TEA-TREE (*Melaleuca linariifolia*)

This has the same common name as the *M. alternifolia*, but is a much taller variety. At one time *M. alternifolia* was described as a variety of *M. linariifolia* before being raised to specific rank by Cheel (while *linariifolia* was classified by Smith). Both varieties are still cultivated for their oils, which are unfortunately often sold under the *alternifolia* name. The main difference between the essential oils from the two varieties is that there is an inverse alpha thujene/alpha pinene ratio – it also has a high cineole content. Otherwise the constituents of the two are quite alike.

OTHER VARIETIES

Black Tea-tree (*Melaleuca bracteata*)
Feather Honey-Myrtle (*Melaleuca thymifolia*)
Lemon-scented Tea-tree (*Leptospermum petersonii, L. citratum*)
Swamp May (*Leptospermum liversidgei*)

The Constituents
of Tea Tree Oil

TEA TREE OIL

α-pinene (2.6%)

α-thujene (0.9%)

camphene (slight trace)

β-pinene (0.3%)

sabinene (0.2%)

myrcene (0.5%)

α-phellandrene (0.3%)

1,4-cineole (slight trace)

α-terpinene (10.4%)

limonene (1.0%)

β-phellandrene (0.9%)

1,8-cineole (5.1%)

γ-terpinene (23.0%)

trans-β-ocimene (slight trace)

ρ-cymene (2.9%)

terpinolene (3.1%)

hexanol

β-caryophyllene (0.1%)

β-gurjunene (0.1%)

aromadendrene (1.5%)

terpinen-4-ol (40.1%)

α-bulnesene (slight trace)

allo-aromadendrene (0.3%)

humulene (trace)

trans-piperitol (trace)

γ-muurolene (slight trace)

viridiflorene (1.0%)

α-terpineol (2.4%)

piperitone

α-muurolene (0.1%)

α-amorphene (trace)

bicyclogermacrene (0.1%)

cis-piperitol (trace)

α-cadinene (1.3%)

allyl hexanoate

ρ, α-dimethylstyrene (trace)

$C_{15}H_{24}$ (slight trace)

α-cubebene (trace)

trans-sabinene hydrate (trace)

α-ylangene (slight trace)

α-copaene (trace)

camphor

α-gurjunene (0.2%)

linalool (trace)

cis-sabinene hydrate (trace)

trans-menth-2-en-1-ol (0.2%)

β-elemene (0.1%)

cadina-1,4-diene (0.1%)

nerol (slight trace)

ρ-cymen-8-ol (slight trace)

calamenene (0.1%)

palustrol (trace)

methyl eugenol (trace)

ledol (slight trace)

cubenol (0.1%)

globulol (0.2%)

viridiflorol (0.1%)

rosifoliol (trace)

spathulenol (trace)

1,2,4-trihydroxy-menthane (trace)

REPRINTED WITH PERMISSION FROM 'THE COMPOSITION OF AUSTRALIAN TEA TREE OIL' BY G. SWORD AND G. L. HUNTER (J. AGRIC. FOOD CHEM., VOL. 37, NO 5). COPYRIGHT 1989 AMERICAN CHEMICAL SOCIETY.[1]

References

TEA TREE OIL

Introduction

1. Cited in S. Drury, *Tea Tree Oil* (C. W. Daniel, 1991), p. 3.

Native Folk Remedy of the Australian Aborigines

1. Captain Cook, *A Voyage towards the South Pole* (an account of his second expedition), Vol. 1 (reprinted 1977), p. 99.

2. T. Low, *Bush Medicine* (Collins, Angus and Robertson, 1991), p. 95.

3. J. White, *Journal of A Voyage to New South Wales* (London 1790); cited in A. B. Cribb and J. W. Cribb, *Useful Wild Plants in Australia*; (Collins, 1982), p. 16.

Early Medical Research Reports

1. E. M. Humphrey, 'A New Australian Germicide', *Medical Journal of Australia* 1 (1930), p. 417.

2. *Australian Journal of Dentistry* (August 1930), cited in Drury, *Tea Tree Oil*, p. 20.

3. A. R. Penfold, 'Some Notes on the Essential Oil of *Melaleuca alternifolia*', *Australian Journal of Pharmacy* (March 30, 1937), p. 274.

Evidence Obtained from Later Clinical Studies

1. Cited in Drury, *Tea Tree Oil*, p. 48.
2. E. F. Pena, 'Melaleuca Alternifolia Oil: Its Use for Trichomonal Vaginitis and Other Vaginal Infections', *Journal of Obstetrics and Gynecology* 19 (1962), p. 792.
3. M. Walker, 'Clinical Investigation of Australian *Melaleuca alternifolia* for a Variety of Common Foot Problems', *Current Pediatry* (April 1972).
4. P. Belaiche, 'Treatment of Skin Infection with the Essential Oil of *Melaleuca alternifolia*', and 'Treatment of Vaginal Infections of Candida albicans with the Essential Oil of *Melaleuca alternifolia*', *Phytotherapy* 15 (1985).
5. R. S. C. Barnetson, in *Australian Journal of Pharmacy* (Oct. 1990).
6. A. L. Blackwell, in the *Lancet* 337 (1991), p. 300.
7. A. Shemesh and W. L. Mayo, 'Tea Tree Oil – natural antiseptic and fungicide', *International Journal of Alternative and Complementary Medicine* (Dec. 1991), p. 12.

Production, Chemical Composition and Quality Control

1. Based on a detailed analysis by Sword and Hunter, 'Composition of Australian Tea tree Oil', *J. Agric. Food. Chem.* 26.3 (1978).

Methods of Use, Safety Data and Storage Precautions

1. A. C. de Groot and J. W. Weyland, 'Contact Dermatitis', vol. 27, no. 4 (1992) cited in *Natural Database U.K. Aromatherapy*, vol. 1, p. 22.

2. R. Tisserand, 'Athlete's Foot', *International Journal of Aromatherapy* 2.3 (1989), p. 19.

A–Z

1. C. W. Olsen, 'Case Studies and Testimonials', in *Australian Tea Tree Oil* (Kali Press, 1989), p. 15.

2. J. Price, 'The Use of Tea Tree Oil in Burn Treatment Products', *Modern Phytotherapy – the Clinical Significance of Tea Tree and Other Essential Oils*, vol. I (proceedings of a two-day conference at Macquarie University, Sydney, Dec. 1 & 2, 1990), p. 56.

3. 'Ti-tree Oil and Chickenpox', *Aromatherapy Quarterly* (Summer 1986), p. 12.

4. Ibid.

5. C. DeYoung (Rockwall, Texas), cited in Olsen, *Australian Tea Tree Oil*, p. 20.

6. Penfold, 'Some Notes', p. 274.

7. Cited in Drury, *Tea Tree Oil*, p. 52.

8. Dr S. Cabot, 'The Use of Tea Tree in Clinical Practice' *Modern Phytotherapy – the Clinical Significance of Tea Tree and Other Essential Oils*, vol. I (proceedings of a two-day conference at Macquarie University, Sydney, Dec. 1 & 2, 1990), p. 4.

9. E. MacNamara (Sydney, Australia), cited in Drury, *Tea Tree Oil*, p. 57.

10. R. Ryan, 'Oil of *Melaleuca alternifolia* Dissolved in Liquid Carbon Dioxide Propellant (Bactigas. TM) Used for the Control of Bacteria and Fungi in Air Conditioning Systems', *Modern Phytotherapy – the Clinical Significance of Tea Tree and Other Essential Oils*, vol. II (proceedings of a two-day conference at Macquarie University, Sydney, Dec. 1 & 2, 1990), p. 70.

11. Cabot, 'The use of Tea Tree', p. 5.

12. *Journal of Allergy and Clinical Immunology* 92 (Nov. 1993), pp. 771–2.

13. See the Shemesh and Mayo study in chapter 3, pages 16–17.

14. B. Moyers, *Healing and the Mind* (Thorsons, 1993).

15. 'AIDS Feature', *International Journal of Aromatherapy* 1.3 (1988).

16. Geoff Searle (Avalon, NSW), cited in Olsen, *Australian Tea Tree Oil*, p. 17.

17. Cited in Olsen, *Australian Tea Tree Oil*, p. 19.

18. Personal letter from D. Sharp to Aqua Oleum.

19. Cabot, 'The Use of Tea Tree', p. 4.

20. Humphrey, 'A New Australian Germicide' – see page 9.

21. Dr P. Balaiche – see page 14.

22. Prof. Anderson – extract from the files of the Museum of Applied Arts and Sciences, Sydney, 1974, cited in Olsen, *Australian Tea Tree Oil*, p. 25.

23. T. Lorette (El Toro, California), cited in Olsen, *Australian Tea Tree Oil*, p. 18.

24. See the reports of Pena, Belaiche and Blackwell, pp. 13, 14 and 16.

25. Penfold, 'Some Notes', p. 274.

The Constituents of Tea Tree Oil

1. J. Agric. Food. Chem. 37. 5. (1989).

Bibliography

TEA TREE OIL

P. M. Altman, 'Australian Tea Tree Oil' *Australian Journal of Pharmacy* 69 (April 1988).

—, 'Summary of Safety Studies concerning Australian Tea Tree Oil', *Modern Phytotherapy – the Clinical Significance of Tea Tree and Other Essential Oils,* vol. II (proceedings of a two-day conference at Macquarie University, Sydney, Dec. 1 & 2, 1990).

B. Barnes, 'The Vaginol Range of Formulations containing Tea Tree Oil', *Modern Phytotherapy – the Clinical Significance of Tea Tree and Other Essential Oils,* vol. II (proceedings of a two-day conference at Macquarie University, Sydney, Dec. 1 & 2, 1990).

—, The Development of Topical Applications containing Tea Tree Oil for Vaginal Conditions' *Modern Phytotherapy – the Clinical Significance of Tea Tree and Other Essential Oils,* vol. I (proceedings of a two-day conference at Macquarie University, Sydney, Dec. 1 & 2, 1990).

I. B. Bassett, 'Tea Tree Gel Controls Acne: A comparative study of tea tree oil versus benzoyl peroxide in the treatment of acne', *International Journal of Aromatherapy* 3.2 (1990).

P. Belaiche, 'Treatment of Skin Infection with the Essential Oil of *Melaleuca alternifolia*', *Phytotherapy* 15 (1985).

—, 'Treatment of Vaginal Infections of Candida albicans with the Essential Oil of *Melaleuca alternifolia*', *Phytotherapy* 15 (1985).

M. F. Beylier, 'Bacteriostatic activity of some Australian essential oils', *Perfumer & Flavorist* 4 (1979).

J. J. Brophy, N. W. Davies, I. A. Southwell, I. A. Stiff and L. R. Williams, 'Gas Chromatographic Quality Control for Oil of *Melaleuca Terpinen-4-ol Type* (Australian Tea Tree), *J. Agric. Food Chem.* 37.5 (1989).

Dr S. Cabot, 'The Use of Tea Tree in Clinical Practice' *Modern Phytotherapy – the Clinical Significance of Tea Tree and Other Essential Oils*, vol. I (proceedings of a two-day conference at Macquarie University, Sydney, Dec. 1 & 2, 1990).

C. F. Carson and T. V. Riley, 'Antimicrobial activity of the essential oil of *Melaleuca alternifolia*', *Letters Applied Microbiology* 16.2 (1993), pp. 49–55.

A. B. Cribb and J. W. Cribb, *Useful Wild Plants in Australia* (Collins, 1982).

P. Davies, 'Ti-tree oil for an adult with chickenpox', *Aromatherapy Quarterly* 12 (1986).

C. Dean, 'The Marketing of Tea Tree for its True Worth', *Modern Phytotherapy – the Clinical Significance of Tea Tree and Other Essential Oils*, vol. II (proceedings of a two-day conference at Macquarie University, Sydney, Dec. 1 & 2, 1990).

C. Dean and P. Daffy, 'A Natural Answer to Acne Dilemma', *Modern Phytotherapy – the Clinical Significance of Tea Tree and Other Essential Oils*, vol. II (proceedings of a two-day conference at Macquarie University, Sydney, Dec. 1 & 2, 1990).

C. Dean and R. Guba, 'Australian News', *International Journal of Aromatherapy* 3.3 (1991).

S. Drury, *Tea Tree Oil* (C. W. Daniel, 1991).

K. Fletcher, 'Colonial Medicine in Australia', *The Herbal Review* (Spring 1988).

J. Fogarty, 'Clinical Investigation of a Tea Tree Oil Preparation for the Rehydration of the Skin in the Lower Limb', *Modern Phytotherapy – the Clinical Significance of Tea Tree and Other Essential Oils*, vol. II (proceedings of a two-day conference at Macquarie University, Sydney, Dec. 1 & 2, 1990).

R. E. Goldsbrough, 'Ti-tree Oil', *Manufacturing Chemist* (Feb. 1939).

Dr O. Hellyer, 'Review of Current Safety and Efficacy Studies on Melaleuca Oil to Approved Protocols', *Modern Phytotherapy – the Clinical Significance of Tea Tree and Other Essential Oils*, vol. II (proceedings of a two-day conference at Macquarie University, Sydney, Dec. 1 & 2, 1990).

V. Home, 'Antimicrobial Activity in Perspective', *Modern Phytotherapy – the Clinical Significance of Tea Tree and Other Essential Oils*, vol. II (proceedings of a two-day conference at Macquarie University, Sydney, Dec. 1 & 2, 1990).

E. M. Humphrey, 'A New Australian Germicide', *Medical Journal of Australia* 1 (1930).

M. Kawakami, R. M. Sachs and T. Shibamato, 'Volatile Constituents of Essential Oils Obtained from Newly Developed Tea Tree (*Melaleuca alternifolia*) Clones', *J. Agric. Food Chem.* 38.8 (1990).

T. Low, *Bush Medicine* (Collins, Angus and Robertson, 1991).

W. L. Mayo, 'Australian Tea Tree Oil – A summary of medical, Pharmacological and alternative health research and writings', *International Journal of Alternative and Complementary Medicine* (Dec. 1992).

Dr H. Merkur, 'The Impact of HPV (Human Papilloma Virus) in Gynaecology', *Modern Phytotherapy – the Clinical Significance of Tea Tree and Other Essential Oils*, vol. I (proceedings of a two-day conference at Macquarie University, Sydney, Dec. 1 & 2, 1990).

K. A. Merry, 'Composition of Oils from *Melaleuca alternifolia*, *M. linariifolia* and *M. dissitiflora*. Implications for the Australian Standard, Oil of Melaleuca – Terpinen-4-ol Type', *Modern Phytotherapy – the Clinical Significance of Tea Tree and Other Essential Oils*, vol. II (proceedings of a two-day conference at Macquarie University, Sydney, Dec. 1 & 2, 1990).

B. Moyers, *Healing and the Mind* (Thorsons, 1993).

G. J. Murtagh and R. J. Etherington, 'Variation on oil concentration and economic return from tea-tree oil (*M. alternifolia* Cheel) oil', *Australian Journal of Experimental Agriculture* 30 (1990).

C. W. Olsen, *Australian Tea Tree Oil* (Kali Press, 1989).

E. F. Pena, 'Melaleuca Alternifolia Oil: Its Use for Trichomonal Vaginitis and Other Vaginal Infections', *Journal of Obstetrics and Gynecology* 19 (1962), p. 792.

A. R. Penfold, 'Some Notes on the Essential Oil of *Melaleuca alternifolia*', *Australian Journal of Pharmacy* (March 30, 1937).

A. R. Penfold and F. R. Morrison, 'Tea Tree Oils', in E. Guenther's *The Essential Oils* (New York: Van Nostrand, 1950).

J. Price, 'The Use of Tea Tree Oil in Burn Treatment', *Modern Phytotherapy – the Clinical Significance of Tea Tree and Other Essential Oils*, vol. I (proceedings of a two-day conference at Macquarie University, Sydney, Dec. 1 & 2, 1990).

J. M. Reece, 'Blooming Business', *International Journal of Aromatherapy* 3.2 (1991).

R. Ryan, 'Oil of *Melaleuca alternifolia* Dissolved in Liquid Carbon Dioxide Propellant (Bactigas. TM) Used for the Control of Bacteria and Fungi in Air Conditioning Systems', *Modern Phytotherapy – the Clinical Significance of Tea Tree and Other Essential Oils*, vol. II (proceedings of a two-day conference at Macquarie University, Sydney, Dec. 1 & 2, 1990).

Prof. R. Sachs, '*Melaleuca alternifolia:* An Estimate of its Potential as a Crop for California', *Modern Phytotherapy – the Clinical Significance of Tea Tree and Other Essential Oils*, vol. II (proceedings of a two-day conference at Macquarie University, Sydney, Dec. 1 & 2, 1990).

R. Setright, 'A Phytotherapeutic Approach to the Immune System and Viral Infections', *Modern Phytotherapy – the Clinical Significance of Tea Tree and Other Essential Oils*, vol. I (proceedings of a two-day conference at Macquarie University, Sydney, Dec. 1 & 2, 1990).

L. Shallcross, 'Ti-tree oil and chickenpox', *Aromatherapy Quarterly* 12 (1986).

A. Shemesh and W. L. Mayo, 'Tea Tree Oil – natural antiseptic and fungicide', *International Journal of Alternative and Complementary Medicine* (Dec. 1991).

I. A. Southwell and I. A. Stiff, 'Ontogenetical Changes in Monoterpenoids of *Melaleuca alternifolia* Leaf', *Phytochemistry* 28.4 (1989), pp. 1047–51.

D. Stewart, 'The Scientific Basis and Clinical Significance of Essential Oil Use in Phytotherapy', *Modern Phytotherapy – the Clinical Significance of Tea Tree and Other Essential Oils*, vol. I (proceedings of a two-day conference at Macquarie University, Sydney, Dec. 1 & 2, 1990).

G. Sword and G. L. K. Hunter, 'Composition of Australian Tea Tree Oil', *J. Agric. Food Chem.* 26.3 (1978).

M. Walker, 'Clinical Investigation of Australian *Melaleuca alternifolia* for a Variety of Common Foot Problems', *Current Pediatry* (April 1972).

Dr L. Williams, 'The Modern Tea Tree Story', *Modern Phytotherapy – the Clinical Significance of Tea Tree and Other Essential Oils*, vol. I (proceedings of a two-day conference at Macquarie University, Sydney, Dec. 1 & 2, 1990).

—, 'Selection and Breeding of Superior Strains of Melaleuca Species to Produce Low Cost, High Quality Tea Tree Oil', *Modern Phytotherapy – the Clinical Significance of Tea Tree and Other Essential Oils*, vol. II (proceedings of a two-day conference at Macquarie University, Sydney, Dec. 1 & 2, 1990).

L. R. Williams, V. N. Home and I. Stevenson, 'The Composition and Bactericidal Activity of Oil of *Melaleuca alternifolia* (Tea Tree Oil)', *International Journal of Aromatherapy* 1.3 (1988).

L. R. Williams, V. N. Home and S. Asre, 'Oils of *Melaleuca alternifolia*', *International Journal of Aromatherapy* 2.4 (1990).

L. R. Williams, V. N. Home, C. Uebergang and L. Stemp, 'Scientific Selection and Cultivation of Australian Tea Tree (*Melaleuca alternifolia*)', paper given at the International Symposium on New Crops for Food and Industry (Southampton, Sept. 1987).

Useful Addresses

TEA TREE OIL

It is important to buy good quality essential oils if they are to be effective thera-peutically. Synthetic perfume oils or dilute products do not have the same poten-cy and cannot be substituted for 100 per cent pure and natural aromatic oils. There are now many brands of essential oils available but the quality control and ethical standard can vary.

Aqua Oleum have many years' experience in the field and provide a wide range of top quality oils at very competitive prices as well as a large selection of virgin-pressed carrier or base oils. They can be purchased from health and whole food stores throughout the United Kingdom, as well as from some chemists. Mail order items, individually formulated products, the 'Essential Oil Catalogue' and further information can be obtained from:

Aqua Oleum
Unit 3
Lower Wharf
Wallbridge
Stroud
Gloucestershire GL5 3JA

Tel: 01453 753555
Website: www.aqua-oleum.co.uk

Aqua Oleum also supply their
products internationally to the
following countries:

Eire
Wholefoods Wholesale
Unit 2D Kylemore Industrial Estate
Dublin 10

USA and Canada
Natura Trading
Box 263 1857 West 4th Avenue
Vancouver
British Columbia
V6J 1M4

Hong Kong
The New Age Shop
7 Old Bailey Street
Central

Norway
Terapi consult AS
Frysjaveien 27
0883 Oslo

Finland
Luonnonruokatukku Aduki Oy
Kirvstmiehenkatu 10
00810 Helsinki

Kenya
Armaan Ltd
PO Box 10118
Nairobi

Taiwan
Grace & Pearl Corporation
6 Lane 97
Tung An Street
Taipei 100

If you want to experience a professional aromatherapy treatment, it is vital that you choose a therapist who has undergone an accredited training. The International Federation of Aromatherapists ensures that its members have attained a recognized standard of practice and provides a list of qualified practitioners throughout the United Kingdom.

For those wishing to further their interest in aromatherapy, the Federation also publishes a newsletter, holds open meetings and can recommend training programmes for individuals wishing to gain a professional qualification. They can be contacted at:

The International Federation of
Aromatherapists (IFA)
Stamford House
2–4 Chiswick High Road
London W4 1TH
Tel: 020 8742 2605
Fax: 020 8742 2606

International Society of Professional
Aromatherapists (ISPA)
ISPA House
82 Ashby Road
Hinckley
Leicestershire LE10 1SN
Tel: 01455 647987
Fax: 01455 890956

Other Useful Addresses

Aromatherapy Organisations Council
PO Box 355
Croydon
Surrey CR9 2QP
Tel/fax: 020 8251 7912

The Institute of Aromatic Therapists
Aromed House
66 Upper Bond Street
Hinckley
Leicestershire LE10 1RS

National Association for Holistic
Aromatherapy
PO Box 17622
Boulder
Colorado 8308–7622
Tel: 1 888-ASK-NAHA
Tel: 1 314 963 2071
Fax: 1 314 963 4454

American Society of Phytotherapy
and Aromatherapy
PO Box 3679
South Pasadena
California 91031

Index

abscesses 27, 39–40
acidophilus 91
acne 14, 15, 16, 28,
    35–6
addresses 114–17
AIDS 25, 67–8
allergies 31, 59, 66, 84,
    89
American Society of
    Phytotherapy and
    Aromatherapy 117
analgesics 25, 44, 76
animal care 31, 78–9
anti-fungal properties 24
anti-viral properties
    24–5
antiseptic properties 8,
    9, 24

applications 23–6
Aqua Oleum 114
Armaan Ltd 115
arnica 42
aromatherapists 116–17
Aromatherapy
    Organisations
    Council 116
arthritis 36–7
Associated Foodstuff
    Laboratories of
    Australia 14
asthma 59
athlete's foot 13, 30, 31,
    37, 92
Atlas cedarwood 71
Australian Aborigines
    3–7

*The Australian Journal of
    Dentistry* 9

babies 31, 43
bacterial infections
    23–4
bad breath 28, 75–6
balanitis 38, 43, 90–1
balsamic properties 26
Banks, J. 4
barber's rash 38, 92
Barnetson, R. S. C. 15
baths 27
Belaiche, P. 14, 53
bellbowrie 99–100
benzoyl peroxide lotion
    15
benzoin 47, 50, 51, 62

bergamot 36, 40, 49, 54, 57, 60, 61, 64, 72
bites *see* insect bites
black pepper 46
black tea tree 100
blackheads 28
Blackwell, Dr 15
boils 12–13, 39–40
borage 80
Britain 116
The British Medical Journal 9
British Pharmaceutical Codex 7
broad-leaved paperbark tree 99–100
bronchitis 40–1
bruises 25, 41–2
bumps 41–2, 79
Bundjalung Aborigines 5
Bungawalbyn Creek 17–18
burns 5, 25, 27, 42–3

cabbage tree 3
cajuput 80, 99, 100
calluses 13
Canada 115
Candida albicans 13, 14, 21–2, 38, 43, 55, 71, 75, 77, 89–91
carbolic acid 8
carbuncles 43–4
cervicitis 13, 71
chamomile 37, 40, 44, 45, 46, 48, 54, 57, 63, 66, 77, 81, 88
Cheel 100
chemical composition 17–22
chemotypes 19
chickenpox 30, 44–5
chilblains 46
children 31, 32
Chronic Fatigue Syndrome 67–8
cineole 18–20, 22, 31, 99–100

citronella 71
clinical trials 12–16
cold sores 27, 30, 48–9
colds 5, 47–8
colloidal oatmeal 46
compresses 27
Considen, D. 6
constituents 101–2
Cook, J. 4
Cordyline australis 3
corns 13, 49–50
coughs 5, 47, 50, 62
cracked skin 51
cradle cap 51–2
creams 30
cuts 25, 27, 30, 52–3, 60, 79
cypress 37
cystitis 14, 53–4

dandruff 29, 55–6
Dead Sea salts 80
dental care 28
deodorant properties 9

dermatitis 16, 31, 56–7
dhobi itch 58, 92
diaper rash 43, 77
disinfectant properties
9, 29, 58–9, 85–6,
89
douches 29, 90
dust mites 56, 59

eczema 16, 56 7
Eire 115
endocervicitis 13
eucalyptus 3, 6, 20, 41,
50, 60, 61, 71, 85
Eucalyptus piperita 6
evening primrose 80
expectorant properties
26

feather honey myrtle
100
feet 89
Feinblatt, H. 12
fennel 37

fever 47, 60–1
Finland 115
fish 79
fleas 79
flu 62–3
fungal infections 13–14,
23–4
candida 38, 43
paronychia 78
skin conditions 9
furuncles 12–13, 39–40

gangrene 9
gargling 28
garlic 48, 54, 63, 68,
72
gas chromatography
20–1
gels 30
genital herpes 63–4
geranium 36
ginger 37
gingivitis 75
glandular fever 68

gomenol 99–100
gout 36–7
Grace & Pearl
Corporation 115
Guenther 20

hair care 29, 65–6
halitosis 75–6
hepatitis 68
herpes 16, 63–4
hives 66
Hong Kong 115
Humphrey, E. M. 9, 52
Hunter, G. L. 102

immune system 24, 25,
67
impetigo 14, 68–9
infections 5–6, 8–9, 13
genito-urinary 29
mouth 28, 74–6
types 15, 21–6
influenza 62–3
inhalation 28

insect bites 25, 69–71, 79

insect repellent 30

The Institute of Aromatic Therapists 116

internal use 32

International Federation of Aromatherapists (IFA) 116

International Society of Professional Aromatherapists (ISPA) 116

The Journal of the National Medical Association 9, 12

juniper 37

Kenya 115

Lassak 20

lavender 19, 36, 37, 40, 41, 42, 43, 44, 45, 46, 48, 49, 51, 52, 54, 57, 60, 61, 63, 64, 66, 69, 71, 72, 73, 77, 79, 81, 82, 83, 88, 93

leeches 91

lemon 37, 60

lemon-scented tea tree 100

lemongrass 71

Leptospermum 3, 5

  L. attenuatum 5

  L. citratum 100

  L. liversidgei 100

  L. petersonii 100

  L. scoparium 4

leucorrhoea 71–2

lice 25, 29, 72–3, 79

lotions 30

Luonnonruokatukku Aduki Oy 115

McKarthy 20

McKern 19

maidenhair fern 6

manuka 4, 5

marjoram 19, 37, 47, 48, 50, 62, 63, 81

masks 30

massage 28–9

Mayo, W. L. 15–16, 48

ME 67

measles 73–4

The Medical Journal of Australia 9, 10

medical research 8–11

Melaleuca 3, 5

  M. alternifolia 3, 5, 13, 17–22, 20, 53, 99, 100

  M. bracteata 100

  M. cajuputi 99

  M. linariifolia 100

  M. minor 99

  M. quinquenervia 99

  M. thymifolia 100

  M. viridiflora 99

melissa 57

meniliasis 13

meningitis 84

Mentha piperita 6

methods of use 27–32

Monilia 16, 43, 89

Morrison, F. R. 19, 20

mosquitos 25, 69–70

mouthwash 9

muscles 29, 76–7

myrrh 51, 80, 82

Myrtacaea 3

myrtle 6

naga sores 92–3

nappy rash 43, 77

narrow-leaved paperbark
    tea tree 3–4, 100

National Association for
    Holistic
    Aromatherapy 117

Natura Trading 115

neat application 27–8

neroli 57

nettle rash 56, 66

The New Age Shop 115

niaouli 85, 99–100

Norway 115

oils 30

oral canker sores 16

paperbark tea tree 3,
    99–100

parasites 9, 25, 91

paronychia 14, 78

patch test 31

patchouli 51

pediculosis 72–3

Pena, E. F. 13

Penfold, A. R. 8, 9, 19,
    20

peppermint 6, 61, 83, 85

pets 31, 32, 78–9

pine 37, 50

plantar warts 94–5

poultices 27

practitioners 116–17

precautions 27–32

pregnancy 31

production 17–22

properties 23–6

pruritis 71–2

psoriasis 51, 80

pustules 16

quality control 17–22

rashes 79

respiratory conditions
    28

rheumatism 81

ringworm 82–3, 92

rosemary 37, 66, 81, 82

safety data 27, 31–2

sage 87

sandalwood 50, 54, 72

sarsaparilla 5, 6

scabies 25, 83

scarring 44–5

Second World War 9, 12

secondary properties 25
shampoo 29
shaving rash 38
Shemesh, A. 15–16, 48
shingles 44, 95
sinusitis 84–5
sitz baths 29
skin care 5, 9, 14, 25, 28, 30, 51, 85–7
Smilax glycophylla 5
Smith 100
sore throats 28, 47, 62, 87
sores 5, 16, 30
splinters 27, 87–8
spots 28, 35–6
Standards Association of Australia 20
sterilization 14
stings 69–71
storage 27, 32
sunburn 88
suppliers 114–15
swamp may 100

sweating 60–1, 89
Sword, G. 102
synergy 21

Taiwan 115
tea trees 3–7, 99–100
Terapi Consult AS 115
therapists 116–17
thrush 13, 14, 38, 43, 75, 77, 89–91
thyme 19, 50, 60, 87
ticks 79, 91
Tinea 16, 37, 57, 82, 91
trichomonal vaginitis 13, 71
tropical ulcers *see* ulcers

ulcers
  mouth 28, 75
  tropical 92–3
  varicose 92–3
United States (US) 115, 117
urethritis 53–4

urticaria 66
usage 27–32

vaginosis 15
vaporization 30
varicose ulcers *see* ulcers
veruccae 94–5
viral infections 23, 24, 67
vitamin C 48, 49, 64, 68
vitamin E 68

Walker, M. 13, 49
warts 94–5
White, J. 5, 6
white tea tree 99
Wholefoods Wholesale 115
wounds 8, 25, 52–3, 60

yoghurt 91

zona 44, 95

Lavender Oil

NATURE'S SOOTHING HERB

Julia Lawless

Lavender is probably the most versatile and widely used essential oil. The scent of lavender instantly soothes and relaxes. Throughout the years, lavender's gentle healing power has helped people with a range of physical and emotional problems. It's one of the few aromatherapy herbs that nearly everybody has access to and it has been a popular healing herb for many hundreds of years.

In 1910, a French perfumer and chemist rinsed his hands in lavender essence and thereby halted the onset of infection, which had developed from a burn. Its renowned antiseptic and sedative qualities continue to make it an essential oil for all the family. It can tackle a range of problems including:

- Headaches and migraines
- Insomnia, depression, stress and anxiety
- Burns, cuts and insect bites
- Muscle aches and strains

Rose Oil

Julia Lawless

Often hailed as the 'Queen of Flowers', the rose has held a prominent place in the mythology of cultures, both in the East and West, for thousands of years. It is widely recognized as a powerful symbol of sovereignty, love, femininity, beauty and spiritual insight.

Today, rose oil is as popular as ever, valued highly for both its perfumery and therapeutic uses and is safe, natural and easy to use. This book reveals how it can be used in the home for a multitude of different purposes including:

- Asthma
- Hangovers and headaches
- Depression, stress and insomnia
- Pregnancy

Rosemary Oil

Julia Lawless

Rosemary oil is one of the three most popular essential oils and is traditionally known for its invigorating and uplifting qualities. It has assorted therapeutic uses and it is often used to help muscular aches and pains whilst stimulating the central nervous system.

Rosemary has a refreshing, invigorating effect on the skin and is most commonly used for scalp rubs and skin treatment.

Aloe Vera

NATURAL WONDER CURE

Julia Lawless and Judith Allan

Aloe Vera is regarded as one of the most remarkable of the 1.5 million botanical species known to man. This practical guide reveals how we can use Aloe Vera for twenty-first century health maintenance.

Find out why Aloe Vera is being hailed as nature's best kept secret. The gel from the fleshy leaves of the plant is rich in vitamins, amino acids and minerals and can be made into juices or lotions for the body both inside and out.